# God Knows
## Caregiving
## Can Pull You
## Apart

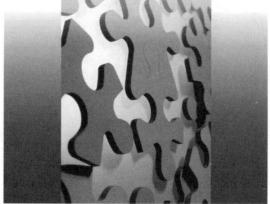

Other Titles in the *God Knows* Series

# God Knows
# Caregiving
# Can Pull You
# Apart

*12 ways to keep it all together*

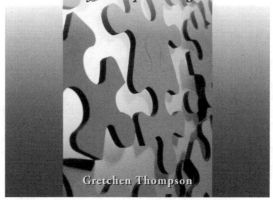

Gretchen Thompson

SORIN BOOKS    Notre Dame, Indiana

As publisher of the *GOD KNOWS* series, SORIN BOOKS is dedicated to providing resources to assist readers to enhance their quality of life. We welcome your comments and suggestions, which may be conveyed to:

SORIN BOOKS
P.O. Box 1006
Notre Dame, IN 46556-1006
Fax: 1-800-282-5681
e-mail: sorinbooks@nd.edu

www.sorinbooks.com

International Standard Book Number: 1-893732-44-4

Cover design by Katherine Robinson Coleman

Cover photography © 2002 Image Source

Printed and bound in the United States of America

*Library of Congress Cataloging-in-Publication Data*
Thompson, Gretchen.
God knows caregiving can pull you apart : 12 ways to keep it all together
/ Gretchen Thompson.
    p. cm.
ISBN 1-893732-44-4 (pbk.)
1. Caregivers--Religious life. I. Title.
BL625.9.C35 T48 2002
248.8'8--dc21

                                                            2002001263
                                                                CIP

# CONTENTS

# Introduction

Joan and Don, both working full-time, had just managed to scrape together a down payment on their first home when two pieces of news came to them almost simultaneously. First, after years of trying and waiting, Joan was pregnant. Second, Don's mother, a widow who lived about fifty miles away, was diagnosed with an illness that would require months of challenging treatment and would also severely limit her capacity for self-care. Not only would she need to move in with them, but someone would need to be home with her during the day. How were Joan and Don ever going to keep up their income, care for her, and prepare for a first baby—all at once?

Nancy, who lived close to her aging parents, began to notice that their forgetfulness and confusion were increasing to the point of being dangerous. They'd already had one car accident driving the wrong way on a one-way street, and sometimes when she visited she found gas burners on or the refrigerator door ajar. She called her brother Mike, and together they researched assisted living facilities. On the day they sat down with their parents to share their suggestions, their father said with fierce determination, "We've lived in this house for fifty years, and I've got news for both of you: we're not going anywhere." How were Nancy and Mike ever going to manage keeping their parents safe while at the same time honoring their dignity and independence?

Jack's wife of twenty-five years had always handled life's ups and downs with a spirit of acceptance and calm that he'd admired and even depended upon. When she began to lose her eyesight, however, she entered into a period of uncharacteristic depression that seemed even more challenging than her vision problems. As her appetite decreased and her sleeping patterns became erratic, he found himself overwhelmed with all kinds of emotions: not only the old familiar tenderness and love, but also deep sorrow, hopelessness, fear, and even anger. How would he ever be able to help his wife—and himself— through this difficult time of loss and change?

Despite what the plots of many a sitcom might imply, life is not always a series of simple happy endings. During the course of our lives many of us—in fact, probably all of us—will face situations in which loved ones become ill or require greater care, situations for which there are no easy answers.

Sometimes these situations slowly creep up on us. Our parents, children, or other loved ones enter into new phases that are simply part of the rhythm of life. Gradually we notice that we're spending whole days driving others from here to there, tossing laundry in and out of the washer and dryer as fast as we can, dropping dishes in our rush to get them washed, and just generally moving along at a demanding pace.

At other times, these situations come upon us quickly in the form of a health crisis or other unexpected shift in daily life. Someone needs care more than ever, and we want or choose to fit that into an already crowded—or overcrowded—schedule.

In either case—slow or quick—caregiving can challenge our old patterns and disrupt our firmly held expectations. We sometimes find ourselves feeling lost in the confusion of figuring out how to adapt and provide. We are forced to make choices we hadn't even anticipated, much less prepared for. Sometimes, simply trying to make it through, we begin to feel pulled in too many directions, almost pulled apart. We exhaust ourselves, deplete our financial resources, or struggle to meet needs and demands that seem as though they'll never end.

Most often, we choose to be there for others because we love or care for them. Ironically, this can make our journey all the more difficult, because in such instances our sensitivity to their wants and needs is heightened, and our desire for their well-being intensified. We feel each challenge more acutely, and our desire to do well often includes a deep but hidden fear that if we don't, the loss will on some level be ours as well as theirs.

However, the very love that can make caregiving seem so painfully poignant is also, often, what can help us through it most of all. The very concern that seems to pull us in so many directions is also what has a true capacity to hold us intact if we learn how to work with it well. For giving care to those we love—no matter how hard it gets—is one of the greatest and richest of all human endeavors. Anyone who chooses to engage in it is not just providing something critically important to another human being, but also inviting into his or her own life an opportunity for profound spiritual growth and deepening of the heart.

Whoever said that the best things in life are easy?

At the core of virtually all religious traditions is a single injunction sometimes known as the "Perennial Philosophy," but no matter what we call it, it amounts to this: *love those near to you.*

In the Jewish and Christian traditions, this injunction is most commonly expressed in the phrase "Love thy neighbor as thyself." Buddhism, Hinduism, Taoism, Islam, and even varieties of philosophy or secular humanism declare a strikingly similar message. This is because love for others is a universal human value. Some would even say it is what holds the world together.

The act of loving another human through caregiving may seem too commonplace, too insignificant in the grand scheme of things, to warrant much attention. Not so.

When Ann Bancroft prepared for a near-impossible expedition that would make her the first woman to reach the North Pole, her friends composed a song for her that began, "Every long journey begins with one step." By the same token, every situation that calls out for human love in action, whatever the scale—be it personal, nationwide, or even worldwide—begins with simple and steadfast gestures of care: one after the other, step by step, person to person. Caregiving is important!

Needless to say, it is easy to love someone else when they are doing well, when they are far away, or any time the conditions are calm and the sailing smooth. The challenge and true test of love is how to express care, how to show it and embody it in our own actions when difficulties arise, when needs increase, when resources are taxed, and when it would be easier to simply walk the other way.

If you're holding this book in your hands, you've probably already chosen to embody this latter version of love, the more challenging kind. Please give yourself some credit for that choice right off the bat. Not everyone has the courage to make it.

Perhaps right now you are thinking to yourself: *Well, sure, I've made a choice to provide care, but how could I do otherwise? After all, she's my mother* or *he's my husband* or *that's my own child; how could I not?*

I understand that it may not feel like a choice for you, but experience tells me that this is more about who you are than about whether the choice truly exists. Through my chaplaincy work in homeless shelters, public programs, and hospitals, I have seen countless individuals for whom there was no one willing to provide care. This is a world and culture in which people really do at times—for whatever reasons— abandon their mothers and fathers, their brothers and sisters, their children, to fend for themselves in the face of life's difficulties. If you are involved in a caregiving situation with a loved one, believe me, you are doing something valuable and something that is not a given with everyone else, no matter how much it may seem that way.

Even a cursory glimpse inside our shelters, public care facilities, and hospital emergency rooms will quickly show you otherwise.

## But How to Keep It All Together?

A great and courageous question! That's what this book is all about. It's for those who have crossed the threshold of "if" in regards to caregiving, and moved on now to the "how" of it.

Each chapter that follows focuses on a different way to "keep it together" while giving care to a loved one.

Included in each chapter are brief explanations about how a particular way might look or work for you, short quotes for inspiration, stories about how others have gone about it, and a number of exercises that you can use to pause and reflect, regroup, and expand your caregiving repertoire.

Because journaling in particular can be such a useful exercise for caregivers, and because its tools (paper, writing utensil) are compact and simple enough to be brought into almost any setting, most chapters will include at least one journaling suggestion. Many caregivers have told me that journaling—writing in a completely non-judgmental way about their lives and having one certain safe place to express their experience in all its complexity—gives them valuable insights that might not be gained as easily in any other way. All exercises, however, including journaling ideas, are only suggestions.

This is a book that need not be rushed through. In fact, it will probably serve you better if you wander through it slowly and thoughtfully, perhaps even in a spirit of well-deserved leisure. It might sit on your bedside table, get tucked alongside a favorite armchair, or travel with you in a purse, briefcase, or satchel. Its quotations and stories are intentionally brief, that they might easily be remembered for inspiration or sustenance at just the right moment. Write them on sticky-notes, if that would help, and put them up on bathroom mirrors or workplace walls. Tell them to others.

Also, you need not read this book from beginning to end. Feel free to pick out the chapter that seems relevant to you at a given time. Chapters are organized in loose priority, beginning with themes that have proven most consistently useful to caregivers, but each of us has a unique way of proceeding. Tailor your reading to fit your needs.

In other words, use each chapter and all that it contains in any way that will help you. The sole purpose of this book is to support you in your caregiving efforts. If reading it becomes yet one more task among many, set it down for another time.

Rachel Naomi Remen, a medical doctor and caregiver of many years herself, says this: that dealing with illness or heightened need "may shuffle our values like a deck of cards. Sometimes a card that has been on the bottom of the deck for most of our lives turns out to be the top card, the thing that really matters. Having watched people sort out their cards and play their hands . . . for many years, I would say that rarely is the top card perfection, or possession, or even pride. Most often the top card is love."

Let the card reshuffling begin, then! May your caregiving be blessed, and graced. And all along the way, may your heart grow in understanding of how important, how valuable, love in the face of challenge really is.

# W A Y   1 :

# Create Time Away

TO BE SOMEBODY, YOU MUST LAST.

*Ruth Gordon*

Parents of premature babies born at Children's Hospital in Minneapolis receive the wonderful service of volunteers called "rockers" while their babies remain at the hospital. Rockers are volunteers who come to the hospital for the sole purpose of holding these tiny babies in rocking chairs or standing beside them in their isolettes, cooing at them, patting them, or singing them lullabies for an hour or two at a time, while their mothers and fathers take a break and get some time away.

The doctors and nurses at Children's Hospital have watched countless parents work through the high-stress caregiving situation of tending to a tiny, premature infant, often while simultaneously worrying about other children back home. They find that time away is critical for parents. It allows them to maintain their resiliency and energy, and consequently increases the odds that their babies will thrive after going home.

Time away for caregivers may sometimes seem like a pipe dream, but I tend to agree with the staff at Children's Hospital: it's actually more a necessity. It can also be one of the thorniest and most challenging issues to figure out and to accomplish.

I'd be rich if I could have a dollar for every time I've heard a caregiver say, "But I just can't get away, not now." However, we need to work with that truth for the sake of all concerned.

One reason it pays to ponder this issue of time away is that in many caregiving situations it emerges in the form of a crisis sooner or later. I remember a friend who took on the role of sole support for her aging mother without developing any plans for alternative care. Her mother required little help in the mornings, but from lunchtime on needed fairly constant attention.

My friend, quite excited over the purchase of her first home, carefully arranged for a morning appointment on the closing date. Her plan was to close on the house, and then drive over to her mother's in late morning.

You can probably guess how this story goes. At sunrise on the day of her closing she got a confused and somewhat desperate call from her mother who claimed to need her immediately. My friend had no idea how serious her mother's request was and had no one else to call for help. She had to make a stressful choice in a very short time.

Actually, she chose the escrow closing. Then she rushed to her mother's side, found her rattled but unhurt, and next developed some different arrangements within about a week. It was easier than she'd anticipated to find others who were competent, caring, and willing to help.

Sometimes, the creation of time away becomes a faith or values issue. Yes, being sole and constant caregiver to a loved one can signal deep devotion. It can also signal a kind of distrust: a fear of asking for help from others. In this sense, seeking time away can also be a hidden invitation to practice trust in others and trust in God.

For example, I was almost incapable of literally handing over my firstborn child to anyone else. It felt absolutely true to me that only I could know his needs and fulfill them. As others—my husband, my mother, my friends—gently but firmly wedged him from my clutches and cared for him tenderly and well in their own ways, I gradually awoke to an unexpected truth: he'd be loved by many different people in his lifetime. Each person who loved him would bring him unique gifts; this monumental task was not mine alone. Maybe it meant I was less important than I'd thought. More significantly, though, it meant that I was less alone and that ultimately I could trust what lay beyond my own meager powers to provide for this child, whose well-being was my uppermost concern.

Aside from being a practical asset and a growth-inducing exercise in trust, the creation of time away is simply an important path to joy and rejuvenation. As one of my hospice patients said to his wife one day, "If you don't get out of here and have a little fun, I'm going to die feeling guilty I made your life more miserable than it ever needed to be. Now scoot!"

Of course not all loved ones have this attitude. But the truth is—no matter what their attitude—time away for caregivers is a necessary part of the journey.

Sometimes, the whole thing reminds me of being in a steam bath. If you've ever taken a steam bath, you know that it is an intense experience in extreme heat and moisture that can be incredibly healing and rejuvenating. However, if you stay in the steam room too long, you become limp and exhausted. The value (not to mention the pleasure) of the experience is greatly enhanced by occasional departures into cooler air or water. So too with caregiving. It's a powerful experience, and has much healing potential for all concerned. And yet without those "cooling dips" of occasional time away, it can end up being detrimental to health and well-being. You will become limp, exhausted, and even sick.

As Ruth Gordon said, the key prerequisite for being helpful to others in this life is simply figuring out how to last, or in other words, survive. Creating time away is at the core of "lasting"—that is, sustaining energy and commitment for the duration of any given caregiving situation.

---

IF YOU THINK YOU NEED A BREAK,

YOU PROBABLY DO.

*The "Web of Care" Website*

## Create Time Away

- Find a relaxing place to sit and write. Allowing yourself to put down whatever comes to you, complete the following sentence in many different ways: "In my life as a caregiver, I . . . ." Try to come up with at least five to ten different ways to end the sentence.

- Next, repeat the process and complete this sentence: "In my life outside of caregiving, I . . . ." Again, write several different endings, naming all the events, hopes, dreams, people, and interests in your life that do not have to do with caregiving. You can use your second list as a reminder of why time away is important, and how you might want to spend it.

- Here are three practical ideas that might help you take time away:

    1. Buy a baby monitor. A monitor allows you to listen to someone without always being right there next to them. Now go and read a good book!

2. Invite yourself on a date. In *The Artist's Way*, Julia Cameron emphasizes how important it is to occasionally "take yourself out" for an hour or two all alone to someplace joyful or fun: an art museum, coffee shop, movie, walking path, or simply a bubble bath by candlelight. Once you've invited yourself on a date, put it on your calendar like any other commitment.

3. Take an imaginary vacation in your mind. A pleasant daydream, although it may last no more than a few moments, does break up the patterns of stress and worry that caregiving can create. One of my friends, the mother of six, had a ball planning the trip to Hawaii she was going to take some day. Using library books and travel agency materials, she took a breather every so often by simply "daydreaming" herself to the shade of a palm tree in Maui. If vacation-imagining doesn't appeal to you, consider trying window shopping or catalog browsing.

- Develop a list of people who can help to relieve you temporarily from caregiving. Brainstorm. Think about friends, neighbors, relatives, volunteers affiliated with hospitals, religious institutions, or nonprofit organizations. Call a few people, explain that you're creating a "back-up caregiving list," tell them why you thought of them, and see what they say. Having been on the receiving end of this kind of call, I can tell you that I was honored and more than willing to help in any way I could.

---

AND ON THE SEVENTH DAY GOD RESTED . . . AND GOD BLESSED THE SEVENTH DAY, AND SANCTIFIED IT.

*Genesis*

# How George Befriended
# Peanut Butter and Jelly Sandwiches

George and I had gone to Arizona every single winter for twenty-three straight years. We started out visiting his sister Evelyn and her husband Jack, but over time we developed quite a cadre of friends there. Family members from Michigan, our home state, grew accustomed to visiting us to get a break from the cold and snow. Arizona really became a second home to us.

George and I have been married fifty-three years, and never spent more than a day or two apart in all that time. He is my best friend, my support, and my sweetheart—about as much a part of me as an arm or a leg! So, of course, when George broke his hip this past year, a part of me broke too. (I think it was my heart.) I could barely stand to see him so frail, and would have done everything on earth to help him. That's actually what I did try to do, in fact: *everything on earth*. Without even reducing my own chores, I tried to add in his, as well as all the duties of a primary caregiver. The things we do for love!

It soon became obvious to me that for this year, anyway, we wouldn't be able to make it to Arizona. It never occurred to me to go there without him. Heavens, it never occurred to me to leave his side. The kids tried to persuade me. "Just go for a little while," they kept saying. "You need the rest. We'll take care of Daddy. One of us will even go with you!"

They were right about me needing the rest, but they had no idea how much my heart just yearned to be right near him.

And then one January morning, as my grandson likes to say, "life happens." We got a distraught call from Evelyn. Jack, who'd had heart problems for many years, had suffered a heart attack just hours before and died. They had no children. She was down there trying to handle this all alone.

Now George and I agreed: I had to go to Arizona. Torn as I felt, I simply had to go for the both of us, even if only for a few days.

The kids promised me over and over that they'd take good care of their father. And even though I knew they meant it, I had a sick feeling all the way to Tucson.

Evelyn met me at the airport. When I gave her a big hug, I could feel her shaking and knew we had made the right decision. She and I spent the next several days calling relatives, planning Jack's service, but mostly reminiscing. Through laughter and tears, we shared a lifetime of remembered stories. I did the best I could to comfort her. I even read, on George's behalf, something he had written to honor Jack at the funeral. George had always seem to be the confident spokesman for the both of us. This time, I stood alone.

It's hard to explain what happened to me on that trip, what I learned, what I experienced. The main thing, though, was probably that loving someone does not always mean being right there with them. Evelyn had now been separated from her husband forever, and yet something special—something deep and true—still existed between them that nobody could have missed. You could just feel her caring for him, and his for her across the greatest divide of all. Of course she grieved deeply and felt his absence. She also felt his presence. And though it was true that she would never hold Jack in her arms again, it was also true that, in a very real way, nothing could separate her from him. Nothing. I thought about that a lot.

I thought too about my own husband back home, in the hands of some very well-meaning children whom I knew could not—no matter how hard they tried—do things for him the way I did. Suddenly, it didn't matter quite so much to me anymore. I saw that George and I one day would be separated by death. And I gained new trust in the sustaining power of our love, which didn't really need to be expressed in every single gesture, every single minute, because our love was bigger than that. It was deeper and stronger.

I'll never forget the day I returned to Michigan. I walked in the door and there was George, on the couch. He was having a tea party with our five-year-old granddaughter Leigh. She had carefully spread her tea set out on the nearby coffee table. Little cups and saucers, toy spoons, a tiny china pot were all carefully arranged there. She had even tucked a napkin under his chin, and was chattering away with him as though he were the best tea-time guest a girl could ask for.

As they talked and laughed, Leigh and her grandfather were feasting together on peanut butter and jelly sandwiches. Indeed, he seemed to be enjoying himself a great deal!

Now I happen to know that George has always hated peanut butter and jelly sandwiches—which makes that moment all the more special to me. Through this experience I have come to trust this far more than before: love knows no bounds; it will always find a way—whether I'm there to make it happen, or not.

*Ruth James*

---

THERE IS THE RISK YOU CANNOT AFFORD TO TAKE, AND THERE IS THE RISK YOU CANNOT AFFORD *NOT* TO TAKE.

*Peter Drucker*

# Janny Draws Upon Time Away

Jeanine, the single mother of a five-year-old, responded to her cancer diagnosis with courageous determination to fight it with all the strength she had. For months it looked as though she would win, but then a devastating relapse put her into bed for what would be months and months of gradual weakening and increasing pain.

Her caregiving support system was excellent, one of the best I've ever witnessed. She moved into the home of her parents, who set aside their own lives to offer Jeanine and her daughter their full care for as long as was necessary. Jeanine's many friends gathered around as well, providing yet another significant influx of daily care and loving company. A hospice team was also brought in, which meant that she had access to specially trained doctors and nurses, physical therapists, dieticians, social workers, personal care attendants, and chaplains. I was her chaplain.

Despite this unusually solid support system, Jeanine's gradual decline was very painful for all that knew her. She was so young and so determined to live. How could this be happening?

Caregivers in situations like this easily become stressed and exhausted, even with the support of one another. There is something especially difficult and draining about dealing with a dying process that seems premature or unfair. Jeanine's mother in particular had an instinctive need to do literally everything she could and found "time away" almost impossible to consider.

The adult caregivers expressed, in addition to all this, a number of worries about Jeanine's daughter, Janny. They were afraid Janny would have the extra difficulty of recovering from the loss of her mother, and they were afraid that nobody could provide Janny the support she was going to need in the difficult time immediately following the death of her mother.

Although I too had deep-felt concerns about Janny, I also noticed that in terms of certain caregiving skills she was extremely gifted—more gifted than her adult counterparts. The greatest of these gifts was her ability to create time away for herself.

Maybe it isn't fair to say that she "created" time away. More accurately, she lacked an adult attention span and simply could not focus on any worrisome situation—even this one—for more than a little while. She frequently took breaks without even being conscious of it. In a completely natural rhythm, Janny would go visit her mother by crawling up on the bed into her arms, then drift out into the backyard to look at the birds and bugs, then settle for a while with her crayons and papers, then return to her mother's arms again.

I began to pay special attention to her drawings and noticed that they too were about "time away" from the oppressiveness of this particular interval in her life. She drew horses that she and her mother used to ride together, and rainbows they had seen. She drew pictures of their dog, their friends, and their home. It was as though she wanted to document not just the illness itself, but all those other scenes, events, and memories that were also part of her relationship to her mother.

Janny taped her pictures in crooked rows all along the wall of her mother's bedroom. Bold, bright, and childlike, they gave literally anyone who glanced at them a little break from the constancy of the illness they all struggled with. No matter how stressed you felt, you could not help but smile at her beautiful, tender gallery.

When the cancer had progressed so much that death seemed imminent, Janny was still drawing, but the pictures changed. She began to draw angels with fluffy white wings and big red hearts. "These are the angels that are going to help my mom in heaven," she would tell me. And then she would surround them with items she thought might be needed: a blue bike for Jeanine to ride, a pair of pretty shoes, bananas, apples, and ice cream cones.

It wasn't that Janny was out of touch with the gravity and sadness of the situation. Her trips to her mother's bed were often tear-filled now, and she asked questions that revealed how much she was experiencing fear. It was just that her drawing of images took her beyond the sheer suffering of the illness. This was an ingenious, if unintentional, form of respite.

One morning Janny told me she was going to draw the whole universe for her mother. I was impressed. "The whole universe! Can you fit it on the paper?" I asked.

"No," she said, giggling at me for being so silly. "I'll use lots of papers and tape them together." And so she began.

First Janny drew the things of the earth: animals, birds, fish, sky, water, grass, flowers, mountains, and cities. Then she moved beyond the earth, and drew the sun, moon, planets, stars, comets, clouds, and meteors.

After a period of concentrated work, she had used up about twenty sheets of paper, and when taped together (I helped with this) they made a huge tapestry. But she wasn't done yet.

Next Janny drew for her mother a whole host of angels. Not just one, but a flock, a full assembly. These we put carefully around the edges.

When we carried this masterpiece into Jeanine's room, she was only intermittently conscious. Janny climbed into her arms as usual, gave her some kisses, told her all about the gift of this special new picture. But when we tried to mount it on the wall, it simply was too big to fit.

"That's all right," Janny said confidently. "Let's put it on Mommy like a big blanket."

And that's what we did. We literally draped over her mother's bed this collage of images depicting the cosmos beyond her illness. And it was under this "blanket" that her mother quietly died a few days later.

Janny, with a child's wisdom, had seemed to understand instinctively that even at a deathbed, there are infinities of other places to remember, to cherish, and to imagine. She taught me more than I can tell about the value of staying in touch with all of life—in all of its multifaceted glory—no matter what.

IF WE DON'T OFFER OURSELVES TO THE UNKNOWN, OUR SENSES DULL. OUR WORLD BECOMES SMALL AND WE LOSE OUR SENSE OF WONDER. OUR EYES DON'T LIFT TO THE HORIZON; OUR EARS DON'T HEAR THE SOUNDS AROUND US. THE EDGE IS OFF OUR EXPERIENCE . . . AND WE AWAKE ONE DAY TO FIND THAT WE HAVE LOST OUR DREAMS IN ORDER TO PROTECT OUR DAYS.

*Kent Nerburn*

# WAY 2 :

# Welcome All Your Emotions

OUR FEELINGS ARE OUR MOST
GENUINE PATHS TO KNOWLEDGE.

*Audre Lorde*

Caring for others—especially those with whom we have an extended history of relationship—can be an experience filled with all kinds of feelings. Many of these emotions—love, tenderness, concern, empathy—are easy to recognize, even easy to welcome into our awareness. Other emotions like frustration, anger, or even rage, disappointment, sorrow, and discouragement tend to be tougher to deal with.

For one thing, we often feel we shouldn't have those kinds of feelings in a situation like this. I've heard many caregivers say, "But how can I possibly be angry at him? He's the one who's sick!" Or, "What right do I have to feel frustrated? She's doing everything she can, and then some."

For another thing, it's easy to forget that *having* an emotion is not the same thing as *acting upon* it. It's one thing, for example, to feel fear: the stomach might flutter; the head might start to ache; the thought process might speed up and become filled with worrisome ideas. But none of these feelings or sensations requires that we actually act upon our fear. What we do with our feelings is truly a matter of choice.

By the same token, feeling angry with someone does not necessarily equate with lashing out at him or her. Nor does feeling discouraged necessarily mean "giving up." Also, feeling happy does not require a straight diet of laughter and song.

Observers and students of caregiving agree that "letting in" or welcoming the whole array of feelings is an important part of what it means to be human and key to healthy caregiving. Why might this have value for us?

In my experience, letting in emotions gives us, in the end, much more wisdom, strength, and resilience as caregivers. The extent to which we can accept others rarely exceeds the extent to which we can accept ourselves, and the practice of embracing all our emotions enhances that a great deal. By embracing all of our emotions, we embrace our humanness. Also, it takes energy to hold back emotions—energy that we may well need for the demands of the journey we face.

Regarding her own experience with feelings of anger, poet Emily Dickinson declared: "Anger as soon as fed is dead; Tis starving makes it fat."

Dickinson meant, I believe, that pretending her anger wasn't there or trying to wish it away actually gave it more "weight" in her life than ever. When she refused to acknowledge her anger, her emotion only found other ways to express or assert itself, ways less obvious, less clear, and ultimately more difficult to work with. On the other hand, when she could simply acknowledge it or give it its day in court, so to speak, then she could decide with a great deal more clarity how to handle all of her feelings.

Emotions are profoundly human, and if we learn to respect and work with them, they can provide us with a magnificent natural notification system about what is happening within and around us.

Perhaps you'd like to learn more about your own emotional messaging system, but are having a difficult time figuring out how. Welcome to the human race! Often, I've found, our body will give us dependable messages about feelings we're experiencing—even when we're not particularly aware of them. Paying attention to our body can be a very useful starting point.

I've noticed, for example, that feelings of stress or tension will often settle in my shoulders and neck, tightening and bunching up the muscles there. When my body feels light all over and is able to glide freely and easily through space, I can trust that I'm filled with joy. Headaches often signal fear or worry. Laughter signals ease. And tears, of course—even when I hold them back—are about sorrow.

Though your body may "hold" your emotions in different ways than mine, paying attention to them can tell you a lot.

The main thing to remember is this: emotions in and of themselves are neither good nor bad. They just are. The more of them we experience, the more alive we are. By welcoming them in, we gain a great opportunity to learn what it is they have to tell us.

Along those lines, perhaps you've heard of Burt and Emma. Neither one of them liked to express emotions much. They hardly ever wept, hardly ever laughed, hardly ever talked about what was going on inside of them. Indeed, they were so quiet about their feelings that when they turned up at the plane ride booth at the county fair, the stunt pilot who took people out for flights was secretly excited. "Finally!" he thought to himself. "At last, some folks who won't scream, holler, and snap at me to stop the ride, or whine and complain about how scared they are. This'll be great!"

Sure enough, through all the loops, dips, spins, and slides, neither Burt nor Emma expressed a single emotion. The pilot, unleashed at last from customer complaint, flew even more daringly, more wildly than he ever had before.

Finally, returning to the runway, he shouted over his shoulder to them, "Now wasn't that the greatest ride you've ever been on? Weren't you scared? Weren't you thrilled?"

After a long silence, Emma made one brief comment.

"Yup."

"When was that?" the pilot asked, eager to hear which of his stunning feats had thrilled her the most.

Her answer surprised him, to say the least.

"Well," she finally said, "I did feel kinda funny back there, when Burt fell out of the plane."

---

LIFE WITHOUT EMOTION IS LIKE AN

ENGINE WITHOUT FUEL.

*Mary Astor*

## Welcome All Your Emotions

- Practice listening to what your body is telling you. Try quick "body-checks" at times when your emotions are more clear to you. For example, next time you're indisputably angry see if you can feel how that is affecting you physically. Also, ask yourself where you can feel a good joke; that's likely where your joyousness settles. Eventually, you'll be able to "translate" in the opposite direction. You'll develop a fierce headache, for example, and know you're frustrated. You'll slip unintentionally from laughter to tears, and realize it's not just a coincidence: you're overstressed.

- Make two lists. In the first, write all the emotions that are most difficult for you. Next, pick just one difficult emotion, and make a game of listing all the different ways you might choose to use it. One woman I know made a list about the feelings of guilt that tended to infuse her caregiving on a daily basis. As you will see, she became more and more playful as she went along. Here is her list:

  1. Put guilt to work; use it as a motivator to get things done.

  2. Have a conversation with my guilt. Ask it where it comes from, and what it needs and wants.

  3. Play guilt all out on the piano—for as long as I want.

  4. Share my guilt (calmly if possible) with the one I'm giving care to.

  5. Share my guilt with a good friend who will just listen and not judge.

  6. Stand in the shower until my guilt washes off.

  7. Introduce guilt to my emotion of self-confidence, and send both of them out the door on a date.

  8. Tickle my guilt (gently, lovingly) until it lightens up a little bit.

  9. Give my guilt a homey space in my big toe, and tell it to stay there until I figure out what to do with it.

---

EVERYTHING IN LIFE THAT WE REALLY ACCEPT UNDERGOES A CHANGE.

*Katherine Mansfield*

# An Act of Courage

When I first went to visit my new hospice patient, James, and his wife, Mae, a strained silence lingered between them that I did not know how to interpret. Speaking with Mae alone later, I learned that she was actually quite angry, on top of that, ashamed, and beneath it, very sad.

At first she was unwilling to talk about her anger to her husband or children, to me—to anyone for that matter. When I told her I thought she'd feel much better getting "it" off her chest, whatever "it" was about, she said something like this to me: "I just have no right to be angry at him. He's *dying*, for God's sake. How could I be angry at a dying man? And yet I am. I'm so angry at him I could scream.

"You see, he was an active alcoholic for over twenty years. When I first married him, we had a very special and loving relationship, but all the time the kids were growing up, he was increasingly undependable and emotionally absent. I got stuck more and more with all of the parenting, and a lot of money problems.

"Last year—for the first time—he went to treatment and got sober. And he stuck with it too! I was so proud of him. We all were. He started going to AA, and got himself a sponsor, and I was just so excited about finally getting him back. The kids were grown, and I could not stop thinking about what a blessing it was going to be to finally regain his love and affection as our retirement years were beginning. I imagined us spending these last years together in some semblance of the caring we had known when we first got married.

"And then, exactly six months—six months!—into his sobriety, he was diagnosed with terminal cancer. I know it sounds crazy, but how could he leave me now, after all this waiting and all this struggle? Why now?

Even though I hate myself for it, I keep having surge after surge of anger at him for deserting me yet again."

Mae was ashamed to welcome in her own emotions, and this was literally silencing her. In fact, it was preventing her from connecting to Stan on a deep level during the precious little time that remained for them.

I sensed that her anger was only on the surface, and that if she could peel it back, she'd find other emotional layers beneath it. I tried to help her discern what the anger was signaling or covering. At the same time, I was deeply touched by both the immensity of her courage and the depth of her determination. This was no casual caregiving situation, and here she was, grappling with all her emotions—not just the easy ones, but the hard ones as well.

"You must love this man very deeply," I said at last.

"But then why am I so angry? Love doesn't get angry! Love is patient and kind. That's what the Bible says anyway. I'm just being a jerk, a selfish jerk."

"Wait a minute, Mae. If you didn't care about the guy, his death wouldn't mean very much to you," I said. "You could just go through this time with a certain distant indifference, and be done with it. In fact, if you didn't care about James, this diagnosis might even be a relief for you.

"Maybe the depth of your anger has something to do with the depth of your love for him, and your sorrow at having to say good-bye. I bet if you found some way to tell him about it, he might even hear it as a compliment."

Mae could see that her anger might well signal how deep and strong her essential caring for him was, but she couldn't figure out how to express it in a way that she'd consider acceptable. Every scenario she imagined seemed whiney, childish, trite, cruel, or pointless.

"Couldn't you just tell him?" I asked. "On a quiet day, maybe, when you're both rested, without raising your voice or anything, you could just tell him how much you struggle with anger—and all kinds of other hard emotions for that matter—knowing that he's going to die after you've finally just gotten him back."

She looked doubtful. "Let me think about it."

The next time I came to visit, the atmosphere had changed entirely. Stan and Mae were calling each other sweet nicknames and acting almost like young lovers with one another, even though he had since been confined to a hospital bed in the living room.

"I had no idea she had that many feelings about me," he confessed, as they spoke together about their recent conversation. "I thought I'd been such a hard man to live with all these years, that she was glad I was dying—just waiting quietly for me to go! But we had it all out. She told me everything, and that gave me a chance to be her real husband again. I promised her I'd try to be there for her in every way, even though we have just a little time left.

"Maybe," he added at last, "what we lack in quantity, we can make up for in quality."

What Stan and Mae reminded me of was that when we don't welcome our own emotions, we give up many of our choices about how to handle them. And when we don't exercise such choices, our loved ones are left to do a lot of guesswork. And then our original intentions—to not hurt them—sometimes become sabotaged.

---

Those who don't know how to weep with their whole heart don't know how to laugh either.

*Golda Meir*

# When the Cork Pops

I am the divorced father of a seven-year-old boy named Sammy, who is the light of my life. I grew up in a home where only one family member—my father—was demonstrative with emotions. Unfortunately, because rage was the emotion he usually expressed, the rest of us spent a lot of time tiptoeing around and trying to keep things calm. None of us, not even my mom, wanted to upset him and get him going.

My dad was under a lot of stress when we were growing up, and I now understand more about some of the reasons he acted like he did at home. But back then, all I knew was that his rage terrified me, and all I cared about was making it go away.

When I grew up and got married, I promised myself there was one thing to which I would never submit my family: that kind of rage. I knew what it was like to walk around in a perpetual flinch, always afraid and on eggshells. That had been a hard and fearful experience for me. I didn't want my own kids to have to go through it.

There's an old song that goes, "If you exorcise your devils, your angels may leave too." That's kind of what happened to me. I was so intent on holding back negative emotions that I ended up holding back lots of positive emotions too. Without being aware of it, I became more and more distant. Everything seemed safer that way. My wife, originally attracted to me by what she thought was a calm and gentle personality, began to tell me more and more about how difficult my emotional absence was becoming for her. And yet, the two of us kept at it anyway. We had Sammy together, and tried our best.

It was my wife who provided most of the emotional support for Sammy. I kept a certain distance. It was a relief for me to learn that I really could control my anger, in a way my father had never managed to. On the other hand, I wasn't much of a father. I worked a lot, and mostly watched TV at home.

When Sammy was five, my wife asked for a divorce. I wasn't devastated because I was just plain numb. Instead of actually allowing myself to feel what that kind of deep rejection was doing to me, I got all logical about it. I found a new living situation, one where Sammy could visit on weekends. I filled up the extra hours of time alone by working more. I read lots of books. You get the picture.

I know now that all that logical thinking was actually a cork that held volatile emotions inside of me so I wouldn't have to deal with them. Sooner or later, that cork just had to blow. Which it did, about six months into the divorce.

One sunny Saturday morning in spring, Sammy was at my place and had a baseball game that day. In my usual detached manner, I was planning on dropping him off at the ball field and going to work for a few hours. We'd had breakfast, gotten him all suited up, and were headed for the door when the phone rang. It was Sammy's coach calling to say that the game had been cancelled. I don't even remember the reason why anymore, I just remember how I reacted.

All I could see was red. I began to shout into the phone. It made no sense, but I couldn't help myself. Blind fury welled up inside too quickly and forcefully for me to hold it back. I had gone crazy. After I had screamed at the coach and made a string of senseless accusations, he—to his credit—hung up on me.

Sammy, who had never seen me like that before, just stood there staring, pale as a ghost, trembling, and blinking back tears. I remember looking at him and hating myself. It was a horrible moment.

I thank God that I didn't strike him or start throwing things around. However, it is completely clear to me that I easily could have. That my emotional rage didn't turn into something more physical was only a matter of coincidence, grace, or dumb luck.

I dropped the phone, and went immediately into my first full-blown panic attack. Suddenly I couldn't breathe. Black terror overwhelmed me. Though the attack itself probably lasted a few minutes, it felt to me like hours. I thought I might be having a heart attack or a stroke.

When the attack had begun to subside somewhat, I immediately called Sammy's mother. She quickly came and got him. Next I called a taxi and went to the acute care clinic attached to our local hospital. I was too afraid to drive.

The road from there has been a gradual journey toward recognizing and dealing with my own emotions, including the hard ones. Learning to live gracefully with panic attacks has meant being far more in tune with my emotional self than ever before. It just doesn't come naturally, and I have had to rely heavily on the help of both professionals and friends.

Unfortunately, there is nothing I can do to erase from Sammy's past all those years of emotional distance or that terrifying Saturday morning. The only thing I can do is keep working at my own emotional health, no matter how hard it seems at times. And I believe deep inside that every minute of the work is worth it.

Every time Sammy comes to visit, every time he freely laughs or cries or stomps his foot to show honest frustration, every time he gives me a big smack on the cheek and a hug, I am reminded again how much my effort is worth it. Slowly—very slowly—I am learning to accept all of my feelings, and all of my self: devils, angels, and everything in between.

*Jim Dodson*

---

I OFTEN WONDER WHY LOVE IS EQUATED WITH JOY WHEN IT IS EVERYTHING ELSE AS WELL. DEVASTATION, BALM, OBSESSION, GRANTING AND RECEIVING EXCESSIVE VALUE, AND LOSING IT AGAIN. IT IS RECOGNITION, OFTEN OF WHAT YOU ARE NOT BUT MIGHT BE.

*Florida Scott-Maxwell*

# WAY 3 :

# Pace Yourself

---

TIME GOES, YOU SAY? ALAS, TIME
STAYS; *WE* GO.

*Austin Dobson*

A common expression—especially among those of
us engaged in giving care to others—is this one:
"Where did all the time go?"

We do this errand, we do that favor; we run here,
stop there for this or that, all the while moving at a pace
both rapid and determined. Suddenly it seems as
though all the time available to us has literally slipped
through our fingers.

Dobson's point is well taken, though. It isn't *time*
that goes anywhere. It isn't *time* that gets lost, spent,
consumed, or wasted. It's *us*. Time will still be flowing
along effortlessly, long after we have come to an
exhausted halt. This is why pacing can be so important.

During her stay in Ethiopia as a Peace Corps
volunteer, my friend Cathy used one of her rare days off
to go mountain climbing. This particular mountain was
known to be challenging, and native guides were sent
along to help her party in case there was any trouble.

Cathy was in great shape physically and had
developed plenty of stamina during the previous
months. As she set out up the mountain with the other
climbers and guides, she was feeling excited,
determined, and full of energy. Her pace was vigorous

and enthusiastic, and she could not understand why the others were going so slowly. They seemed to be walking in slow motion. And this was not just the other climbers, the guides seemed to plod along as well!

When she suggested that she move on ahead at her own more rapid pace, the lead guide smiled somewhat mysteriously and told her to go right ahead. His only request was that she stay on the path, so that if they caught up with her, they'd be able to find her again.

Two miles or so later, Cathy, who had almost sprinted along thus far, found that her calves were beginning to ache and her breath was becoming increasingly short.

A half mile later, she was feeling even more winded, and her whole body hurt. She slowed her pace a little bit to accommodate this unexpected sense of exhaustion. A half mile after that, she was too tired to take another step, and sat down on a rock to wait for the others.

Sure enough, around the bend they came, chatting with one another and looking full of energy. Their pace was just as it had been earlier—slow and steady, one foot after the other. Cathy, still too tired to go on, had to wait for them as they slowly trekked to the summit, took a look at the breathtaking view, and headed back down again.

There is something to be said for pacing, especially when the journey is uphill.

Sometimes it seems that when we have more to do, when the role of caregiving is added in with our other life roles, the best solution is to simply "go faster" and try to accomplish more than we ordinarily would, by increasing or at least maintaining our normal pace. Especially if we're used to achieving what we set out to achieve, this is the most natural impulse in the world.

Cathy was a smart woman. She wasn't trying to deceive herself about what she could or couldn't do.

She was just new to mountain climbing. Having grown up on the plains of the Midwest, she didn't have all the information she needed about what this kind of travel demanded. Her guides certainly could have told her to slow down, but perhaps they knew that experience would be her best teacher.

Caregiving can be a kind of mountain that many of us flatlanders have not experienced before. Chances are, it will require us to learn some new rhythms and techniques, some new ways to pace ourselves.

Pacing becomes important in caregiving situations because the consequences of exhaustion can be serious. Cathy only needed to sit down on a rock for a while. This had few consequences for her or for anyone else. Not seeing the view at the summit was a loss, but not a heartbreaking one. Exhaustion in caregiving can be more troublesome, leading to major disruptions. Work schedules can come to a halt because of illness or stress. Children can lose out on attention. Sometimes more help needs to be brought in at greater expense and inconvenience.

It pays to pay attention to pacing!

Of course, nobody can learn a new pace instantly or perfectly. This makes it inevitable that we'll push ourselves too fast at certain times, and go more slowly than we need to at others. There is great value, however, in noticing our pace, and working with it.

---

SOMETIMES YOU WONDER HOW YOU GOT ON THIS MOUNTAIN. AND SOMETIMES YOU WONDER, "HOW WILL I GET OFF?"

*Joan Manley*

# Pace Yourself

- Take more careful notice of your present pace in caregiving. Tune in on it intentionally. It's amazing how much we sometimes forget to do this. The following list of questions to ask may help:
  - Do you feel ready to collapse when it gets to be mid or late afternoon?
  - Do you struggle to wake up in the morning?
  - Are you feeling like each day contains more things to do than you can possibly accomplish?
  - Are you skipping meals?
  - Are you forgetting tasks or responsibilities that you usually remember?
  - Do you feel irritated by events or concerns that used to roll right off your back?
  - Have you stopped seeing or even talking to friends you used to spend time with regularly?
  - Do you ever find that, even when you *do* have a chance to rest, you're too restless to utilize it?
  - Do you experience any symptoms such as heart palpitations, grinding your teeth, outbreaks of arthritis, or headaches?
  - Are you increasing your use of alcohol, tranquilizers, or sleeping medications?
  - Do you ever forget what you're doing or who you're talking to?

Any "yes" answers here are signs that you may need to pace yourself more slowly. Pushing yourself along, at this point, may only deplete your resources even more.

- This is simply a bit of practice in prioritizing. Early in the day, make a list of all the things you want to get done. Now skim through the list a few more times:

  - Put a star next to two or three items that are *absolutely essential*.

  - Put someone else's name next to any item you can *delegate*.

  - Put a check by two or three items that could *wait until tomorrow*.

  - Just for practice, draw a line through one or more items that you can actually *skip altogether*.

- Kim Lund suggests another prioritization exercise: Make a list of the day's tasks in prioritized order from most to least important; then cut the list in half and throw away the bottom half.

- See how many things you can touch only once. This strange-sounding advice comes from my mother-in-law Barbara Ferguson, who learned somewhere along the line that her frenetic pace resulted from skimming from task to task without making final decisions about any of them. She was setting too many things aside for later, only to have to deal with them over and over again. Try these kinds of changes:

  - When you pick up your mail, sort through it one time only. Standing near a wastebasket, throw out many pieces you would have once saved. What doesn't get tossed can land in one of two bins: *Answer* and *Pay*. Go through these piles also, but only once a week.

  - Instead of setting the garbage down by the back door, carry it out immediately.

  - Put dishes straight into the dishwasher, instead of setting them in the sink.

Add your own creative ideas.

- Put affirmations in creative places. A friend has this
message taped inside his desk drawer at work: "You
become a hero by staying at the office about as much
as you become a car by sleeping in the garage." Use
these affirmations, or be on the lookout for ones that
suit your own situation best. The search alone gives
you a great excuse to visit Chinese restaurants
regularly, hoping for the right fortune cookie!

---

THERE IS MORE TO LIFE THAN
INCREASING ITS SPEED.

*Mohandas K. Gandhi*

## Donna's Story

---

I remember being a young mother with two children
in diapers and having a full time job teaching
learning-disabled children in the public schools. There
were days my pacing went wild, days I would race like
crazy from dawn to dusk and still never get it all done.

My teacher's aide, Donna, herself the mother of
five, would watch me race, gently put her hand on my
shoulder, and say, "Take a deep breath now! You'll
never get through this if you don't slow down."

I could never understand what she meant. How
could I get more done by slowing down? It seemed
counterintuitive, even a bit nonsensical. And yet, she
was a tried and true caregiver and her load was clearly
greater than mine was: more children and just as many
working hours. So how did she do it? She quite
dependably seemed rather cheerful, patient, kind, and
content.

Finally I asked her! And then she gave me the gift of this story, which moved me deeply and also changed my perspective about trying to do too much too fast.

"When I had my first baby," she began, "I got tremendous joy out of keeping her in cute little ironed dresses, washing her diapers myself, and making her food out of fresh produce in the blender. I wanted so badly to be the best mom ever, and I had the time to do it. It was great!

"When our second came along less than two years later, I wanted to do the same for him. I noticed that it was a little harder, though, taking care of two little ones so carefully. Some nights I was almost reeling with exhaustion.

"When the third baby was born, I forced myself to pick up my pace even more, and basically tore around every day trying to get everything done. It was becoming less and less fun, but I was so determined. It never occurred to me that I needed to do anything differently.

"Well, then came the fourth. I was maxed out. I had no time for myself at all. My appearance went to pot, my social life didn't exist, and I was more exhausted and unhappy than ever."

Donna paused, as if to consider how much she really wanted to tell me. Then, seeming to confirm something within her heart, she continued.

"To tell you the truth, when I learned I was pregnant with the fifth child, I was just overwhelmed. I couldn't see any way to go on. I actually drove my car to a bridge at the edge of town one night and sat there thinking what it would be like to just go through the guardrail and end this crazy rat race for good.

"I prayed to God to help me, and tell me what to do. Instead of getting instructions to end everything, though, I got just one thing—an idea—but it was a good idea. It slowed my pace almost immediately, and has served me well ever since."

Needless to say, by then I was rapt with attention. "What was the idea?" I asked, like a desperate miner in search of gold.

"It was pretty simple," she warned me. "It was just this: love the first child first."

"What?"

I didn't get it.

"Well, here I was with four children going on five. When I tried to love them all at the same time, I just ran around like a chicken with my head cut off. That way, none of them really got what they needed—my wholehearted attention—and I just exhausted myself trying.

"But when I remembered to love the first one first— to pay full attention to the one who needed it most at the moment—I found that the others weren't so fussy as you'd think! They watched me, saw a woman calm and competent, and knew that if they just waited, this same calm and competent woman would eventually get to them too.

"Of course I had to give some stuff up. You can't love them well, one by one, if you take on crisply ironed clothes for all five as your top priority. But my love for them really *was* the most important thing to me—I'd just lost track of what that actually meant.

"As time went along—and this was the best surprise of all to me—they began to copy me the way children do with their mothers, and started paying wholehearted attention to each other!

"Thank God I drove away from that bridge. Our youngest, Michelle, is a beautiful child, and she gets everything she needs from me—or someone else— eventually. Our life wouldn't be complete without her.

"So that's what I learned. Hardly rocket science, even though I had a heck of a time getting to it. Love the first one first with all your heart, and slowly but surely, everything else will fall into place. You don't need to race, you don't need to rush. Just do it."

NOTHING CAN BE MORE USEFUL TO
YOU THAN A DETERMINATION NOT
TO BE HURRIED.

*Henry David Thoreau*

## One Pebble at a Time

It probably wasn't even six months after my dad had died. My mom was still pretty much of a wreck. He hadn't left behind enough to support us, so she had plenty of worries about money, keeping the house, and finding a better job. In some ways, my little sister Elizabeth and I were left to take care of ourselves. She was only seven at the time, and I was thirteen. Life just gets hard sometimes.

It was a Sunday morning, and we were all lined up in our pew at church, still trying to get used to Dad not being there, feeling the harsh pain of that, but also needing friends and community around us for support. Church was awfully good that way. Someone was always giving Mom a hug or asking how she was doing. Elizabeth and I got a lot of extra love and attention there too. It helped a lot.

Anyway, on this particular Sunday, our pastor was talking about faith and what it took to sustain it over the long haul. That was an important theme for us right then, which may be why I remember what he said so clearly even now, twelve years later.

He was saying how our faith life needed to have a good steady, even pace—not too rushed, not too slack—in order to keep going. The story he told us was about this man who went walking with his three children. Every morning, they'd go together to this mountain, pick up one pebble, carry it to the far side of a nearby river, and set it down again.

These walks were slow and relaxed. They involved long looks at the sunrise, plenty of fresh air, green fields, and flowers. The man, on these walks, taught his children everything he knew about living a good life: treating others kindly, being responsible, and so forth.

Well, the man's children grew to love this simple tradition so much that when they grew up they taught it to *their* children: walking to the mountain, picking up one pebble, carrying it across the river, and setting it down again. Their children, in turn, taught it to *their* children, and that way the tradition got passed down through generation after generation.

At this point in the story, the pastor paused, looked out on all of us, and finished the story with this line that I bet I'll never forget: "Until it became so," he said, "that the mountain was moved."

I'd heard that expression "faith enough to move mountains" before, but in my imagination that had always meant waving some kind of magic wand or experiencing some kind of miracle with lots of thunder and lightening, so that the mountain got moved in one amazing instant. But this was a different kind of faith: slow, steady, and dependable. And it was another kind of way for faith to move mountains: one pebble at a time.

After church that day I lay on my bed thinking about it. I thought about the mountain of trouble facing our family, and what it would take to move it. If we tried to take on everything at once, we'd fail, that was for sure. The answer had to be something different: something dependable and steady, something that took just a little bit of faithful effort every day.

I lay there thinking for a good long time. I got out some paper, and a pencil with a good eraser. I worked with my calculator, wrote out lots of numbers, juggled them around, and thought some more. Then I went to Elizabeth's room, and told her my idea. Even though she was only seven, she understood it pretty well.

By dinnertime, my heart was pounding. I felt filled with a kind of faith I'd never known before.

"Guess what, Mom," I said, as she was dishing up meatloaf and peas. "One thing you don't have to worry about anymore is getting Elizabeth and me to college. We've figured out how to pay for that ourselves."

My mother almost froze, her spoonful of peas hanging in mid-air. "Oh, Ned," she said, concern written all over her face. "You shouldn't be worrying about that kind of thing. That's my job, to figure that out. You should be going to school, and having fun with friends, and playing baseball—not giving up your childhood to earn money."

Elizabeth couldn't hold back any more. She blurted out excitedly, "No, Mom, we did figure it out, and we won't have to give up our childhood! And it's gonna be fun, because we're gonna save pop cans!"

My mom smiled—a little indulgently, I thought— but after all, the scheme did sound pretty harebrained.

If you hadn't worked the numbers, that is.

In our state at that time, you could get a two-cent refund for every pop can you brought in to the recycling center. We drank pop, and so did our friends and neighbors. You could also collect pop cans at school functions like my baseball games and Elizabeth's drama club performances. Probably the people at church would help us out too.

I'd calculated it pretty carefully. If we turned in enough pop cans each month, and if we put our earnings in a savings account with interest, and if we just kept at it long enough, we'd have enough money to go to college. Not some private liberal arts college far away, maybe—but definitely our own state university. And it would only take a little bit of effort each day. The main thing would be to keep our faith—keep it steady and dependable, like the minister said.

I showed my mom the pad of paper with all the numbers on it. At first she looked like she was going to start crying, but instead she said something like, "Ned, your father would be so proud of you." And then—this is the best part—she smiled a little bit. And even though we'd only solved a small part of the total problem, she seemed to keep smiling a little bit more each day, after that.

I'm twenty-five years old now. I graduated from college two years ago, and Mom says I ought to go on and become a pastor. Elizabeth will start her freshman year at the university this coming fall.

Pop cans paid for my education, and they'll pay for hers too. I know it sounds crazy, but it really did work. In fact, if I have kids of my own someday, I'll teach them how to do it, just like Elizabeth and I did.

The other night on a TV show, someone made a joke. "How do you eat an elephant?" they said. "One bite at a time!"

I know about that.

How do you get to college?

One pop can at a time.

How do you move a mountain?

One pebble at a time.

How do you live faithfully? One slow, steady, well-paced, deliberate and faithful deed at a time.

*Ned Blakely*

---

FOR EVERYTHING THERE IS A
SEASON; AND A TIME FOR EVERY
PURPOSE UNDER HEAVEN.

*Book of Ecclesiastes*

# WAY 4:

# Watch for Hidden Blessings

VERY OFTEN WHAT YOU REAP IS, IN
THE WAY OF SMALL MIRACLES, MORE
THAN YOU CONSCIOUSLY KNOW
YOU HAVE SOWN.

*Faith Baldwin*

Perhaps you've heard of the Divine Couple of the Hindu tradition, Shakti and Shiva. Even though they occupied the far-off heavens, they tended with great compassion to the goings-on of those on earth.

One day Shakti saw a poor beggar struggling along the rockiest of paths, a man made weak with hunger and hopelessness. She turned to her beloved and whispered, "This one we must help. His heart is kind, and he yearns with such sincerity to avoid stumbling."

Shiva glanced down and watched for a while as well. "No, I don't think we should help him yet," he replied. "He does not look ready to receive our help."

"But we must!" came Shakti's response. "Here, take some of my jewels, put them in this earthen sack, and set the sack directly in his path so that he will find it and be able to buy food for himself. Please."

Shiva, with no little amount of hesitation, did as she had asked him, placing her jewels just around the bend of the very road he trod.

The man, stumbling along exhausted and sad, was lost in thought about his troubles. Turning the bend, he saw something large and bulky in his path. "Ahhh, the largest rock yet, in this endless road of rocks and sorrow," he muttered to himself.

Taking great care so as not to stumble, he stepped over Shakti's bag of jewels, and continued upon his way.

Of course, not all rocky roads contain hidden bags of jewels and not all challenging situations contain hidden blessings. But some do, and we are more likely to notice them if we are on the lookout.

I cannot say exactly where hidden blessings come from. That's part of their mystery. I do know, though, that they often await the open heart and mind, and the discerning eye.

I experience them as signposts of hope along any given journey. They usually do not provide us with major solutions or escape routes. More often they function as sources of encouragement or comfort and can be tremendously helpful in terms of keeping us energized.

The man in the story was looking for trouble, and indeed, trouble was all he could find. He was a good illustration of that old expression, "If you only have a hammer, everything in the world starts to look like nails."

Likewise, if any of us is willing to lift our eyes up off the road and glance around a bit, it is surprising what we can see. The search for hidden blessings does not require a major personality overhaul or reversal of direction. It is more about shifting the angle of one's perspective—just ever so slightly.

My friend Michael illustrates this subtle shift of perspective by telling another story, the Sufi tale of Nasrudin—one of my favorites.

Nasrudin, riding along on his donkey, was smuggling something across the border, but nobody could figure out what it was. They repeatedly searched his backpacks, his pockets, and his boots—every possible hiding place—and were never once able to figure out his trick.

At last, then, they were forced to simply let him be.

Years later, after Nasrudin had become a wealthy old man, one of his friends grew bold enough to ask.

"What were you smuggling across the border all that time?"

Nasrudin turned to his friend and smiled.

"Donkeys . . . I was smuggling donkeys," he quietly replied.

To find a hidden blessing is not about self-deception, nor is it about blind or foolish optimism. It involves honest acknowledgment of what is happening, but then too a willingness to go beyond that, in order to see what may lie around the bend.

Because as a caregiver you are likely facing some situations that are by their very nature difficult or challenging, you might find these strategies useful for keeping your eyes open.

First, *remember that you can't see everything at once.* We as human beings simply lack an omnipotent perspective. We can't know all there is to know about even our own circumstances, no matter how aware we try to be. If we look at the front of a house, we can't see the back of it at the same time.

A second strategy: *Practice "looking at the glass both ways."* Every glass that stands half-empty also stands half-full. Which half of the glass have you focused on so far? Can you add to that wisdom and insight by focusing on the other half as well?

And then a third helpful strategy: *Smuggle in a "donkey" or two yourself.* One sure way to experience life as infused with hidden blessings is to "smuggle them in"—as it were—yourself. This practice has the added advantage of bringing unexpected delight to others.

Maybe you have no time to cook. Is it possible to enjoy TV dinners by candlelight? When was the last time you feasted on spray cheese? Or ordered a gigantic and delicious pizza with everything on it, making sure to include enough slices for leftovers?

Part of the nature of blessings—hidden or otherwise—is that they are bestowed upon us, they come to us uninvited. But just because you can't make a blessing happen, doesn't mean that you can't prepare your heart and soul for one to come along, recognize it when it does come, welcome it into your life, and put it to good use.

---

Each morning we are born again. What we do today is what matters most.

*Jack Kornfield*

## Watch for Hidden Blessings

- Give yourself some quiet time. Let yourself settle into a mood of openness and receptivity. Reflect upon your caregiving situation. Ponder—and then write down—what you are *sure* about. Make a list. Are you sure of the diagnosis? Are you sure of the physical needs that require attention? Sure of the schedule you must tend to, the demands upon your day? These sure details comprise the real road upon which you walk. The details are definitely there, beneath your feet, no doubt about it.

Now make a second list. What are you *unsure* about? What remains open and unpredictable? What might you learn from this situation? How might you grow? How might relationships evolve or change? What has become possible that was impossible before? What will happen tomorrow, or in a week, or a month? Hold on to this second list. It will often describe for you the terrain in which hidden blessings can be found, nestled like unhatched eggs in the wilderness.

- Play with water. Begin your day by filling a glass with water to the midway point and setting it by the sink. Imaginatively, then—or better yet, literally—put a little water in every time you experience a blessing, and take a little out every time you experience a disappointment. Do this for a few days, and you'll develop a sense of whether you're experiencing your life as "draining" or "filling." If the glass is generally brimming by evening, take it as a sign you're in touch with life's blessings. If it's empty, let it be a warning that something about your caregiving situation needs to change before you are seriously depleted.

- Bring blessing to another. Sometimes, when you give, you have less. Other times, when you give, you have more. Concrete things—things like money, clothes, food—are often in the former category. True kindness, on the other hand—compliments that you *really* mean, for example, phone calls you *really* want to make to friends, or surprise visits with those who *truly* appreciate you—are often in the latter. Think of what you might do today that would simultaneously bring blessing, energy, joy, to another and to your own self. Then go do it!

WHEN GOD AT FIRST MADE MAN,

HAVING A GLASS OF BLESSINGS

STANDING BY;

LET US (SAID HE) POUR ON HIM ALL

WE CAN.

*George Herbert*

## Annie's Story

One day last year, walking down the corridor of a local hospital, I came upon a room with a closed door, outside of which stood about fifteen teenagers. One young woman in particular seemed to be bent over with grieving. The others—seeming only a little less sad themselves—were nevertheless gathered around her to offer comfort and encouragement.

This was an unusual scene along these normally quiet and empty hospital hallways. I visited with them long enough to understand.

The girl, whose name was Annie, was waiting for the doctors to finish speaking with her father who had been hospitalized yet again for complications that were part of his chronic illness. Her mother was in there too, Annie said, and her friends, well, they always came along like this. This particular relapse, she added, had seemed more serious than the others.

"How long has your dad been sick?" I asked.

"Ever since I was a little girl. I guess as long as I can remember."

"And how is it that you have so many friends here to help?"

"Oh, they're here to help me for sure," she explained, "but they love him too. It's like he's everyone's dad." Her friends nodded in silent agreement.

I thought of all the fathers I knew who barely had enough time to spend with their own children, much less a group of friends this size. I wondered how this had come about.

"So how did he get to be 'everyone's dad' like that?"

"Well, he's been at home to meet me after school every day ever since I can remember," Annie explained. "Lying on the couch, that is, but even so, always ready to give me a hug and ask me how the day went.

"So when I started to bring home friends, he would always ask them how their day went too. And pretty soon, they all got to know him."

"We've watched a million movies with him," another kid chipped in, "and he'll talk to us about just anything. Annie's dad is really cool. And he's really funny. And he's always nice to us."

I knew I was witness to a hidden blessing. Annie's father had clearly traveled a long and hard road with his illness, and probably his whole family had too. It seemed to me that he'd been unable to work, and that his wife had likely been gone from dawn to dusk most days earning family income.

But what he had given back to his daughter and her friends from his spot on the couch was a gift of immeasurable proportion. He had given them something that in our fast-paced society is almost priceless: steadfast, dependable affection from a concerned adult.

The next day, I passed by that corridor again, and the kids were all gone. The room was empty as well. I checked with a nurse. Annie's dad had died. But I knew that the memory of his kindness would live on for years in the lives of his daughter and her friends.

---

WE RECEIVE FRAGMENTS OF HOLINESS, GLIMPSES OF ETERNITY, BRIEF MOMENTS OF INSIGHT. LET US GATHER THEM UP FOR THE PRECIOUS GIFTS THAT THEY ARE, AND RENEWED BY THEIR GRACE, MOVE BOLDLY INTO THE UNKNOWN.

*Sarah Moores Campbell*

## Not by Bread Alone

---

While visiting her elderly parents, Nancy noticed that both of them had ceased eating well and become dangerously underweight. She contacted their doctor, and subsequently made a difficult decision to hospitalize both of them—on separate units, it turned out—until their conditions became more stable.

Her parents had not spent one night apart in over fifty years. Her mother in particular grieved the separation so deeply that hospital personnel feared it might be as detrimental to her health as lack of nutrition.

Every time Nancy visited, all her mother could say was, "But why have you separated us? I need to be with him, and he needs me. I miss him so." Understandably, this was very hard to hear, and even harder to solve.

One day in the midst of this, Nancy followed an impulse and spent the afternoon combing her parents' home for old photographs. On a number of poster boards, she mounted picture after picture of her father beginning with his boyhood, progressing through their wedding day, the births of all their children, hunting trips, holidays, every memorable event, great or small.

The next time she went to her mother's hospital room, she and the nurses set these up all around the bed almost like bouquets of flowers. Her mother was so relieved that she began to weep. Gently she reached out and touched the old photos one by one, almost as though this tactile gesture would bring her closer to her loved one.

Perhaps she could not be with him for a time, but she could at least spend the long days ahead remembering their life together and all of its special moments. The photographs in themselves gave her new will to recover. She had truly needed some reminder of him nearby, and it had been given her. Nancy's part in all of this had been but a moment of thought, and an afternoon sorting through boxes in the attic. It was a simple thing, and yet in its own way, a stroke of genius.

Most of life's circumstances can be made easier by the arrival of unexpected blessings. We as human beings have both a capacity to receive them, and—perhaps more than we know—a capacity to find them, seek them out, and allow them to heal us.

---

SO IT WAS EITHER A MIRACLE—OR
MAYBE IT WAS MORE OF A GIFT, ONE
THAT REQUIRED SOME ASSEMBLY.

*Anne Lamott*

# WAY 5:

# Find Fellow Travelers

WE DO NOT WALK INTO THE
KINGDOM OF HEAVEN ONE BY ONE.

*Mary Parker Follett*

Fellow travelers—those who understand your experience and will walk alongside you in it—can be tremendously helpful to caregivers.

Perhaps you've heard the tale of the woman upon whose household fell a great many difficulties. An unexpected illness struck many members of her family, leaving her with much to do and much to worry about.

Fearing that she would not be able to bear the weight of this, she went to the wise man who lived in the woods outside her village and asked him if he might work a cure, and lift at least some of these troubles from her home.

He listened carefully to all that she said without speaking a single word. It was only when she had spent herself in explanation, that he replied kindly, "I believe I truly can help you with this. But in order for me to do that, I will need you to bring me a mustard seed from the home of someone whose life is far more trouble-free than yours. You'll need to find a family at least somewhat free of suffering. As soon as you do that, bring me a seed from their home. We'll proceed from there."

Greatly relieved, the woman hurried back to tell her family of this hopeful news. And beginning the following morning, she began to visit the other villagers in search of the special seed.

At the first house she visited, a woman answered the door leaning heavily on a gnarled cane. Her limbs were bent and sore, her pace slow. "Mine is not exactly a home free of suffering," she said, after listening to her visitor's needs. "I am crippled, as you can see, and I am also trying to care for my husband, who is bedridden there in the back room. But please, come in for a little cup of tea. Rest yourself for the journey ahead."

The woman, after gratefully accepting this gesture of hospitality, continued on her way.

At the next house she visited, the young man who answered the door was dressed all in black. After listening carefully to his visitor's request, he said, "I'm afraid I can't help you. You see, my wife and I recently lost our first baby. Even though the funeral was some weeks ago, our hearts are still so heavy that we would never be able to provide you with a seed like that. But please, come in for a little while. You must be tired from all your walking. Besides, my wife would love a visitor."

The woman, after spending some time with the man and his wife, continued on her way.

She visited the third home, then the fourth and fifth, until eventually she had been to every home in the village. Still she held no mustard seed in her hand, for not one family she'd met could claim freedom from suffering. In every family, in every home, she heard about some form of strife, loss, or struggle.

She returned to the wise man. "I never did find a seed to bring you," she said, "but for some strange reason I am feeling so much better! Even though my neighbors all had their share of trouble to bear, so many of them were kind to me, and so many were understanding."

"Perhaps what you've gained instead of the seed," he said quietly, "is the knowledge that you are not alone."

She looked startled at first, but then said, "I do believe that's it!" And with a renewed sense of gratitude and hope, she returned to her own home once again.

The challenges of caregiving are sometimes compounded by a deep and disturbing sense of isolation. And once we begin to feel all alone—once we sense that no one else could ever understand quite what we're going through—we stop reaching out. Needless to say, this in turn increases our isolation. And yet, there is tremendous power in journeying with others who understand.

When my husband first began to lose his eyesight as a result of long-term diabetes, his needs, and his capacities—indeed his whole life—changed slowly but dramatically. This meant that my role as his wife also shifted. Caregiving needs increased and so did isolation. It was a gradual process and a subtle one, almost unnoticeable at first.

At first the old friends with whom we had enjoyed playing doubles tennis for years stopped calling. One of the foursome could no longer play! How were they to connect with us now? Gradually, other friends—not out of any kind of meanness, so much as confusion about how to handle his loss of eyesight—invited us over less and less.

The less they called, the more I assumed that isolation was part and parcel with our new situation. I could have called them and said, "Don't worry about whether he can eat spaghetti blind, your friendship is more important to me—to us—than all the plates of spaghetti in the world!" Strange as this may sound, such phone calls simply didn't occur to either of us. Furthermore, I didn't know a single other spouse who was dealing with long-term effects of diabetes, and I didn't know how comforting and encouraging a "traveling friend" might really be.

By sheer luck, grace, or coincidence, I happened to meet a woman about my age who was the mother of a child with autism. Though her caregiving responsibilities were quite different from mine in an outward sense, she understood me deeply and from the heart when it came to my internal struggles. Because she knew from experience how truly lovely it could be to have someone to call, she invited me to give her a ring whenever I felt sad or in need of a bit of encouragement. She didn't know my husband—as I didn't know her daughter—so she had no preconceived ideas about what I was experiencing. She was just there to listen, support, and offer cheer as needed. I came to depend upon her and care for her deeply, and before long could return to her some of the gifts she had so freely given me. She was an "insider" to the world of extended caregiving. She knew that to laugh sometimes could be tremendously life-giving and rejuvenating. I never had to worry about being judged by her. She was open recipient of both my laughter and my tears.

A traveling companion is a precious thing.

---

Hearts that never lean, must fall.

*Emily Dickinson*

## Find Fellow Travelers

- Research information on local caregiving support groups. Check with your local hospitals, medical clinics, churches, or even the yellow pages. Some groups are designed for a specific situation—Alzheimer caregiver groups, for example—and other groups are designed to support you in caregiving situations of all kinds. Often these groups are led by trained professionals and include a lot of good solid information, as well as the camaraderie of others; sometimes, they are self-run.

- Dare to share more with others about what you're going through. In other words, risk being a little bit more open with your story.

- Be open to connections from unexpected places. Sometimes, we are blessed with understanding companions from the most surprising places. One of my co-workers, caring for a wife with a brain tumor, found deep comfort in conversations with a veteran from the Vietnam War who worked down the hall from him. The war had made this man quite wise about handling irrational situations. He was able to be a traveling companion of the best kind.

- Give a little of yourself, even though you feel stretched already. One certain way to receive encouragement, hope, or companionship is to give it.

- Read books by other caregivers. Granted, the conversation in such cases is one-sided, but books can and do connect us with others who understand when we're not quite ready for something more.

- Pause for a while. With pen or pencil and paper near at hand, close your eyes and think about who you would most like to talk to right now about your life as a caregiver. This could be a "real living person" like a friend or relative, but it could also be a beloved grandmother or grandfather who has died, a famous person you admire, a fictional character whose perspective or advice you'd trust—even a saint, or some other wildly imaginative conversation partner!

- Picking up your paper, begin a conversation with this conversation partner. If you could talk to her or him right now, what would you say? Write it down. Then skip a line and allow your pen to write out the partner's response. Of course you have to make this up—let yourself! Quite often, when we love or revere someone or something, we have much better access to what they might tell us than we suspect. It's just a matter of allowing ourselves to focus in on it. Let the conversation go back and forth, until it has come to a natural end. Then ask: What insights have I gained, that weren't accessible to me before? What wisdom came my way?

---

IT SEEMS TO ME THAT TRYING TO LIVE WITHOUT FRIENDS IS LIKE MILKING A BEAR TO GET YOUR MORNING COFFEE. IT IS A WHOLE LOT OF TROUBLE, AND THEN NOT WORTH MUCH AFTER YOU GET IT.

*Zora Neale Hurston*

## Connie and Janet's Story

---

My two cousins, Connie Hanson and Janet Pelto, had finally managed to help their parents move into an assisted living facility, when first their father and then their mother began to show serious signs of dementia. The loss of one parent to dementia is devastating enough, but the loss of two is almost unimaginable for many of us.

Within a relatively brief period of time, these sisters managed to move their parents out of their home of thirty-odd years, settle them in a lovely apartment attached to a nursing home, transfer them again one after the other into dementia units, and observe their parents both experience loss of recognition and many bodily functions.

Connie and Janet are in some ways as different as night and day. Connie, who lives out of town, is detail-oriented and highly dutiful in her role as first child, and knows how to make things run as smoothly as possible. Janet, who lives in town, shies away from working on details and much prefers focusing on the big picture. One could almost assume that such different siblings, under the stress of this kind of struggle, might become critical of one another and impatient with one another's styles of functioning. And yet, when I asked them what it was that helped them most through this caregiving crisis, they responded with simultaneous clarity, "My sister."

Connie remarked, "I remember one day when we were clearing out the house, and we found at least twenty—heck, maybe even thirty or forty—little slips of paper in Mom's desk, with my aunt's phone number written on every single one! Clearly, Mom was having memory problems before we knew about it, but forty slips with the same phone number on them? It was unspeakably sad, in one way, but it just struck me at that moment as the funniest thing on earth. Who else but Janet could possibly have understood? Who else could have known that I wasn't laughing at Mom, but just plain laughing? Even now, looking back, I'm still not all that sure what exactly was so funny. But at that moment, we understood the situation—and each other—perfectly."

Janet, smiling at the memory, added, "I remember how much I hated all the financial and legal details I was supposed to be handling through this transition. I didn't like it. I wasn't very good at it, and I kept forgetting what I was supposed to be doing. And yet, I was the one living near Mom and Dad, so I kept thinking it was my responsibility.

"It would have been so easy for Connie to get mad at me—especially since she loves to keep things in good order—but she never judged me. She just kept saying, 'Do what you can, and try not to worry. We'll get through this eventually.'"

As it turned out, Connie and Janet arranged matters so that Connie handled most of the technical details from out of town, using the telephone and occasional trips to keep everything straight. Janet, for her part, kept a clear overview from nearby. This relieved a tremendous burden for both of them.

And the two sisters found hidden gifts in this extraordinarily challenging caregiving situation. Before, they had been "regular sisters," quite different from one another, though caring enough from a distance. Now, having been through this together, they both knew a great deal more about how much they truly loved, respected, and trusted one another.

---

LIFE WITHOUT A FRIEND IS DEATH WITHOUT A WITNESS.

*Rose McCaulay*

# Lydia and the Cockroaches

I will never forget Lydia, a young mother I met one year while helping with community organizing in a large city. Along with many other women about her age, she lived with her children in a housing complex at best poorly maintained by an absentee landlord. Most of these women, like Lydia, were both working full-time and raising their children alone. At the end of a day, exhaustion was common and frustration high, especially when the elevator was broken or the heat malfunctioning. It's much harder to be attentive to a crying infant after carrying groceries up eight flights of stairs—at the close of a long workday.

These women did not know one another well. Each of them expended all the time and energy they had on their immediate families. They probably assumed that occupants of the neighboring apartment units, as tired as they were, would have little to offer in terms of help or support.

Until the cockroaches arrived, that is.

One spring, the building became overrun with cockroaches. There were cockroaches in her children's cereal boxes, cockroaches slithering out from between dinner plates in the cupboard, out of the margarine dish. No matter what Lydia tried—roach killer, boric acid, shoe slamming—she could not get rid of them. More and more they enraged her, becoming almost a symbol for everything difficult in her life that she could find no way to overcome.

Lydia called her landlord numerous times and also the health department. She knew that there were health regulations about cockroaches, but—call upon call—she could find no one willing to listen to her and come through with a helpful solution.

One night, dozing on her couch before the ten o'clock news after the children had been put to bed, she had a brainstorm.

The next day, for the first time, she began going from door to door, confirming with her neighbors that they too were having a terrible time with the roaches, and explaining what she thought might finally work to get rid of them. By the end of that week, her brainstorm had been refined, improved, and put into motion by a number of enthusiastic neighbors.

One woman took the biggest cockroach she could find to her temporary secretarial job. She stuck it in the copy machine, blew the image up, and made several copies.

Another woman drafted a press release that began: "Cockroaches to protest at landlord's home." The press release featured a story about the cockroaches at a certain inner-city address who had become so sick of the humans interfering with their lives that they'd organized a march and protest rally to take place at the landlord's own home. The date and location were clearly identified.

Lydia herself attached the huge cockroach pictures to the press releases and sent them to every major newspaper in the city. Almost immediately local reporters began to phone.

The children were set to work at a special task: catching cockroaches. For the first time, many of them learned one another's names as they scoured the building with mason jars and kitchen pots, collecting thousands of roaches—all ready to "march."

One of the mothers had borrowed a van. They headed to the landlord's house. By the time they got there, the press was waiting for what would make a great lead story on the evening news.

Lydia, flanked by newfound friends and neighbors, lined the children up along the sidewalk in front of his lawn, all of them ready to release the roaches from their various jars and pots in the event a march was necessary. Then she gave her interview, telling of conditions in their rental unit, telling of the roach-infested hallways, kitchens, and bedrooms that were becoming more and more impossible to inhabit.

The press, of course, wanted the landlord's comments. Though he refused to come out of his house, he did promise to solve the problem immediately if these women and children would only take their cockroach march away from his neighborhood.

Within days, Lydia's apartment building was free of cockroaches. Also, the feeling of the place had changed considerably. Strangers had become traveling companions. Each woman had seen for herself how much could get done when efforts were combined. People said hello to one another in the hallways and traded babysitting tasks.

No doubt about it, a seismic shift had taken place. Such is the power of having a true traveling companion or two.

---

IT GOES ON ONE AT A TIME, IT STARTS WHEN YOU CARE TO ACT, IT STARTS WHEN YOU DO IT AGAIN . . . IT STARTS WHEN YOU SAY WE AND KNOW WHO YOU MEAN, AND EACH DAY YOU MEAN ONE MORE.

*Marge Piercy*

# WAY 6:

# Educate Yourself

---

DO NOT WEEP; DO NOT WAX
INDIGNANT. UNDERSTAND.

*Baruch Spinoza*

Life is full of fascinating information. The other day, a scientist friend told me something I found astounding: A typical cloud is capable of holding about one hundred tons of water. One hundred tons of water! This means that even just one of those fluffy, weightless-seeming wonders is heavier than about two hundred automobiles. Now how could that be? This information certainly altered my perspective on clouds.

Often, that is precisely what information does: It alters our perspective. It alters it by expanding perception, sharpening its accuracy, and affirming its already-existing intuitive wisdom. For all these reasons, gleaning as much information as possible can be useful to caregivers.

As a woman whose husband and son both have diabetes, for example, I love receiving—every single week—an e-mailed diabetes newsletter for lay people and another newsletter for professionals and researchers. They don't cost me anything, and they keep me updated. Despite my general lack of computer skills, I was able to locate both newsletters by simply typing the word "diabetes" into the little box on the screen that says "Search," and then pushing the "Enter" button. *Voila*—an excellent source of information!

Once we begin searching for information that is helpful, the information comes to us much easier. An odd phenomenon can happen in life: As we hone in on what we're asking, information we might not have noticed before becomes more evident. Perhaps this is because the asking itself helps us to focus on what we're looking for. Or maybe the cosmos is just question-friendly!

No matter. Education—the gathering of new information, fresh data, different perspectives—has helped many of us along in our caregiving roles. In fact, at times we have been called to not only take in information but, for the good of all concerned, to dispense or spread it among others as well. This is often because, as L. E. Landon says, "Whatever people in general do not understand, they are always prepared to dislike."

One of the most striking stories about the need for education in recent years was the story of Ryan White, a teenager from Indiana. You may remember Ryan's story because his was one of the first publicized cases of AIDS. Ryan, who had dealt with hemophilia all his life, was diagnosed with AIDS in 1984. Hemophilia often requires blood transfusions, and during one of these transfusions the AIDS virus entered Ryan's system.

After Ryan had spent some initial recovery time at home, he felt ready to go back to school. Like any teenager, he was getting restless apart from his friends and activities. When his mother called to set up his re-entry into the classroom, however, she was told to call back after spring break. When she did so, she was told that, because of his diagnosis, he would not be allowed to return at all.

In the ensuing months, Ryan and his family were exposed to a great deal of unnecessary humiliation. Not only was he was repeatedly blocked from re-entering school, but the parents of other students actually picketed his home to make it publicly clear that he was unwelcome there. The local Board of Health tried to put a quarantine sign on his home. County officials tried to make him a ward of the court, as though his condition was caused by neglect or abuse on the part of his supposedly unfit parents.

This nightmare of social ostracism was largely about lack of information. Ryan himself is said to have told reporters at one point, "Well, they're just trying to protect their own kids, like my mom's trying to help me." This was true, but the problem was, it had no basis in accurate knowledge.

What the other parents did not have was any kind of substantial information about HIV/AIDS and how it is transmitted. If they had learned that HIV/AIDS can only be transmitted in a few ways, mostly involving intimate mingling of bodily fluids, their fears about the virus invading the immune systems of their own children through casual contact would have been reduced. Their lack of education cost unspeakable suffering for a boy and his family.

Gaining information can help us deal with our fear and grief. Passing information on to others can be empowering, invigorating, and also constructive for the surrounding community. The truth is that all of us can stand to learn something by increasing our knowledge of one another's circumstances. This increases our compassion and our wisdom.

Education comes in many forms: from a conversation that picks up one well-placed comment or bit of information, a one-hour session at a nearby school, a brief article in a local newspaper, a few moments spent with a book, or a heart to heart talk with a friend.

We can count on at least two pieces of good news as we begin to educate ourselves about an illness or caregiving.

First, we will find wonderful resources available. Sometimes the information we need will be financial or legal. Sometimes it will be medical. Sometimes the information will be familial in nature, having more to do with relatives and their opinions, preferences, or assessments. Sometimes, it will have to do with insurance or other resources that can increase quality of care. No matter what the informational need is, there are usually a number of ways to find it and process it.

The second piece of good news is this: It's never too late to start learning. Even if you have experienced difficulties in caregiving due to lack of knowledge and information, a new day dawns. There is always time to learn.

Don't give up. Education—the gathering of relevant knowledge—can only translate into more effective and capable caregiving in the end.

---

THE MOTTO SHOULD NOT BE:
FORGIVE ONE ANOTHER; RATHER,
UNDERSTAND ONE ANOTHER.

*Emma Goldman*

## Educate Yourself

- Make a "Wisdom Wish List." Ten to fifteen minutes spent in quiet reflection can be an invaluable start to building a useful knowledge base. Imagine that a wise teacher stands before you. This "wise one" is capable of answering literally any question you might ask about your caregiving situation. The person's sole intent is to help you improve your situation.

- What would you like to ask this person of wisdom? Write down your questions. If none come to you, dwell for a moment on each of the following areas of caregiving, and see if this helps you to be more specific: legal, financial, familial, insurance-related, medical, community-resource related, psychological, spiritual, practical, emotional. If your list of questions is long, put an asterisk by the three most important ones of all.

- Now close your notebook or tuck away your list. Let the "wise one" congratulate you on your good work and then depart from your imagination. Allow yourself to rest for a bit amidst a real sense of accomplishment. Answers can never precede questions. You may have just completed the bulk of the work around self-education.

- Explore the library. Useful books abound on many specific caregiving situations, and sometimes a librarian or reference system can lead you right to them.

- Search the Internet. A lot of websites not only have information pages, but also boards for posting messages and chat rooms. This means you can ask questions anonymously or have e-mail conversations with others in your shoes, in addition to locating useful, relevant information. Exploration on the Internet can lead to amazing connections and research studies.

- Ask. Medical doctors, religious leaders, lawyers, nurses, and pharmacists all possess different kinds of valuable information. Count on them. And don't underestimate the word-of-mouth search methods that often exist among networks of friends and relatives.

- Visit a bookstore. Bookstores carry the latest books on a given subject, ones that may not have yet found their way into the library systems.

---

WISDOM IS THE PRINCIPAL THING;

THEREFORE GET WISDOM: AND WITH

THY GETTING, GET UNDERSTANDING.

*Book of Proverbs*

## If Mike Had Only Known

Claire Berman, in *Caring for Yourself While Caring for Your Aging Parents*, shares many poignant and informative stories about the risks of not having enough information. One story, about a man I'll call Mike, described an individual with an extraordinarily generous heart.

Mike had worked in his father's family business for several years. As his father grew older—and became more confused—Mike cared for him with extraordinary dedication by helping him increasingly with the business, as well as visiting him daily at home to make sure his basic needs were met.

Mike and his wife cooked for his dad and did his laundry. They shopped for his groceries and helped him clean. They shoveled the snow in winter and mowed the lawn in summer. In short, they helped in every way they could.

His father, never particularly easy to get along with, grew more and more unpredictable and difficult—some might even say cantankerous. As Mike began to see that the business was at risk, he asked his father a number of good questions about financial and legal details in order to assure its overall success. His father, in turn, brushed Mike off with a number of vague assurances that the business would eventually be left to Mike and that for now everything was "fine."

Mike knew he needed more information. He was wise to ask for it. However, when his father dismissed him, Mike let it go, operating on a loose assumption that somehow everything would work out in the end. After all, it was hard on a good day to challenge his father's directives or opinions. As his dad grew more difficult, it just didn't seem worth it.

Unfortunately, everything was not—as Mike's father claimed—"fine."

His dad had been secretly complaining more and more to Mike's out-of-town brother about how Mike and his wife were smothering him in their caregiving, tender and loving as it was. Over a period of months, significant rancor developed on Mike's brother's part, even though Mike had no clue about what had been going on.

I would like to tell you that this is not a true story, but in fact it is. Mike was completely blindsided at his father's death. His out-of-town brother inherited the bulk of the business, told Mike to expect no role in its future operation, and expressed only contempt for the years of caregiving he and his wife had provided to their dad.

Needless to say, Mike's loss at that moment was devastating. He was forced to part with a father he had trusted and loyally cared for, a business he had spent the majority of his adulthood building, and his relationship with his brother whose caregiving load he had uncomplainingly carried for years.

Even a cursory glance at his father's will, or the briefest of honest conversations with his brother, for that matter, would have given him some invaluable information.

Life isn't always so predictable, and neither is caregiving. Generous hearts aren't always enough. Be encouraged, as one with a generous heart, to take good care of yourself. Learn!

---

KNOWLEDGE ITSELF IS POWER.

*Francis Bacon*

## Gaining Knowledge in New (and Old) Places

Both of my parents were born in Laos. My family came to America when I was a little girl. I speak both English and Hmong and have always known how to move back and forth between these two cultures, though they are so different that at times this is difficult.

As a young woman I married Chris, who is also a first-generation Hmong American, and the two of us have always lived with my mother-in-law, according to Hmong tradition.

When our second child Laura was six months old, she developed a very high fever. I was the financial administrator in a nearby church at the time, and usually left Laura in her grandmother's care during the daytime. We thought that maybe she was coming down with chicken pox, and that it just needed some time to work its way through.

When the fever was still high after several days, though, Joyce—our church secretary and a good friend of mine—strongly urged me to take Laura to the doctor. When we took Laura into the clinic that evening the doctor was very concerned, and she ended up in the intensive care unit of the nearest children's hospital.

Poor Laura! She was so tiny to be hospitalized and separated from the rest of us. My mother-in-law spent most days with her, and Chris or I would spend evenings and nights there, just so she wouldn't have to be left alone.

After a few days, the doctors in the hospital came up with a diagnosis for Laura: meningitis. They thought that it was being caused by a bacteria, but they wanted to do a spinal tap, to find out more.

We listened carefully, and knew we would have to make a very hard decision. Spinal taps were risky, but there was also a risk involved in neglecting to do one. We began to wonder if there might be, in addition to the understandings of American medicine, wisdom from the Hmong tradition that could help us, and help Laura.

Hmong and American medicine are very, very different. Most Hmong believe that each human being has a Spirit that comes to earth with it for a time. If the Spirit has unmet needs or wants, or if It wanders off somehow and becomes separated from the body, then illness can result. Whereas many Americans will turn to a medical doctor when they are sick, traditional Hmong will turn to a *shaman*.

A shaman, though as highly revered as any doctor among those he or she serves, is trained in a completely different way. A shaman's special skill is learning what the Spirit needs, and then developing a strategy for providing it—usually through rituals, acts or ceremonies that most Americans would find unimportant.

We were extremely fortunate because our primary physician at the children's hospital understood both systems.

First, she had become an American doctor, trained in a well-known medical school. At one point she went to Thailand, to help in the retention camps there, and learned enough Hmong to be able to speak many of its dialects fairly well. She also learned to appreciate the ways of the shaman.

As we discussed the risk factors of a spinal tap for Laura, she openly encouraged us to utilize Hmong tradition, and consult a shaman to see if it might help.

In the end, we decided to use both American and Hmong ways, to bring our baby back to good health. The hospital provided us with a great deal of excellent medical expertise, but we decided against the spinal tap. Instead, we brought in a shaman who determined another kind of diagnosis: that Laura's Spirit was dissatisfied with her given name. In a special ceremony, he helped us to discern a better name, and then give it to her.

Laura began to recover almost immediately. Within a short time her fever had dropped, and she was able to come home from the hospital.

I do not know if her recovery can be credited to the one system of knowledge, or the other. Probably each played a part. Most of all, though, I am extremely grateful that I was encouraged to seek thorough understandings of both traditions, different as they are from one another.

To this day, our family continues to use both Hmong shamans and American medical doctors. From the former, we constantly gain education in the healing ways of our own cultural heritage. From the latter, we learn a great deal about what Western medicine has to offer. Because we have chosen to open our hearts and minds to a variety of wisdoms, we consider ourselves doubly well informed, and doubly blessed!

*Song Thao*

WE HAVE A HUNGER OF THE MIND
WHICH ASKS FOR KNOWLEDGE OF
ALL AROUND US, AND THE MORE WE
GAIN, THE MORE IS OUR DESIRE; THE
MORE WE SEE, THE MORE WE ARE
CAPABLE OF SEEING.

*Maria Mitchell*

# WAY 7:

# Be Open to the Gifts Your Loved One Has to Offer

---

TRUE SERVICE IS NOT A
RELATIONSHIP BETWEEN AN EXPERT
AND A PROBLEM; IT IS FAR MORE
GENUINE THAN THAT. IT IS A
RELATIONSHIP BETWEEN PEOPLE
WHO BRING THE FULL RESOURCES
OF THEIR COMBINED HUMANITY TO
THE TABLE AND SHARE THEM
GENEROUSLY.

*Rachel Naomi Remen*

With all the complications of caring for others, we might be tempted to start believing that we are the ones doing all the giving, and the person we care for all of the receiving. What could they possibly have to give to us, when we are most likely the healthier one, the stronger one, or the one simply expected to provide a majority of care?

I spoke with a woman the other day who had grown dangerously drained from caring for her mother who suffered from dementia.

"And what does she give you back?" I asked.

"She can't give anything back," came the reply. "She used to be a great mom. She took such good care of me, but now she talks and I don't know what she means. She seems to be in some different world, and half the time, she doesn't even seem to recognize me." Tears welled up in her eyes as she was reminded of all that she had lost.

Sometimes I have this kind of conversation with parents as well. Their kids are young, they say, and still in need of so much. What could a dependent five-year-old possibly be expected to give?

Indeed, being the recipient of gifts from those we care for often seems out of reach. Isn't expecting *anything* just a set-up for disappointment? So why even hope for what is unlikely, if not impossible?

There are two reasons. First, being open to another's gift promotes human dignity all around. Second, being open to receiving gifts back honors that which is often most mysterious and holy about our bonds to one another. Let's look at human dignity first.

Think about your own life. Have you ever been in a relationship in which you were expected to do all the listening, while others did all the talking? How did it feel? What did it suggest to you about your own capacities? Did it make you feel stronger, or weaker? Larger, or smaller? More capable, or less so? More valued as a human being, or devalued?

The truth is, a steady diet of receiving—in this case, taking direct help from others—is often difficult. It can be painfully diminishing, even exhausting. For you to expect nothing more of a loved one than that they receive what you have to offer them, can put them in a cramped and powerless position. Even if your loved one has dementia or is only five years old, giving whatever they can to you enhances their dignity as human beings and affords them a life-giving role in the grand scheme of things.

I remember the elderly woman confined for weeks and weeks in a special hospital bed, flat on her back.

She had to be fed in such a way as to allow for little head or neck movement. Her children, who had never seen their typically resilient mother in such a condition, were some of the most attentive caregivers I had ever met. They brought her fresh flowers every day and helped the hospital staff feed her, and they read to her for hours on end. Rarely did they leave her alone.

One day, the woman asked one of her daughters to please bring her some yarn and knitting needles from home. Her daughter forgot and came the next day without them. The nurses and I watched her requests for knitting needles go unheeded for about a week. It wasn't that her children were inattentive, but they were so focused on what they thought she needed to receive that they overlooked what she had to give.

Finally, her primary nurse brought in a pair of needles and some yarn from her own home. Immediately, this woman began knitting from flat on her back. By the time I came to visit later in the day, she had finished the first tiny pair of mittens and was beginning to work on the next. Her work was very beautiful, the stitches even and snug.

When I asked her who the mittens were for, she said with a gleam in her eye, "They're for the children! My church group knits mittens for children in our neighborhood who need them every Christmas. Because of being here, I am so far behind! I promised I'd have ten pair ready by December 1, and I just hate the thought of any children having cold hands.

"When I'm done with that," she added, "I'll start making a sweater for each of my grandchildren. I have three, and they're all as sweet as can be."

This woman had gifts to offer the world, flat on her back or not. And her gifts included not just knitting, but an abundance of wisdom about how to endure difficulty well. Being able to fulfill her obligations and help others was important to her dignity.

If it is truly more blessed to give than to receive, then we as caregivers have a moral obligation to enhance and celebrate all the ways those in our care can give, no matter how that manifests itself. Being open to the gifts of loved ones is important for another reason as well: it honors the potential and the sanctity of our bonds with one another.

The tearful woman mentioned earlier, who could not imagine receiving anything from a mother with dementia, left our conversation with something to ponder. The next time I saw her, she had grown aware of a gift she received from her mother at every single visit, a gift that could have easily gone unnoticed. It was the gift of loving touch.

Her mother, whether seeming to recognize her or not, began every visit in the same way. She reached out tenderly and grasped her daughter's hand or wrist. Simply put, love really did continue to flow from mother to daughter, long after words had failed. To at last understand this was, for the daughter, a great comfort.

Caregiving is mysterious. While it may often seem like nothing more than "a relationship between an expert and a problem," as Remen has said, it can be a great deal more. Our task is to remain open to the "something more." We are called to do more than just give, give, give to loved ones. We're also called to receive gratefully from them whatever they might knowingly or unknowingly offer to us.

---

AS LONG AS WE THINK DUGOUT CANOES ARE THE ONLY POSSIBILITY—WE WILL NEVER SEE THE SHIP, WE WILL NEVER FEEL THE WIND BLOW.

*Sonia Johnson*

# Be Open to the Gifts Your Loved One Has to Offer

- Breathe deeply and take yourself back in time. Remember one of your early achievements: how you tied your own shoes, fed a pet, went to school, read a book, or hit a baseball. Remember how it felt to have gained that particular power in the world. Describe in writing both the incident itself and your feelings about it. Now write about how the adults in your life responded to your achievement. Were they proud or were they unaware, so that the achievement went unnoticed? Were they encouraging? Or did they somehow diminish you? Think about your present caregiving situation, and ask yourself: Am I still living by the lesson of how my achievements have been received? Do I want to?

- Ask someone for a favor—any person, any favor: butter from the neighbor, a back scratch from your toddler, breakfast in bed from your teenager, a $10 loan from your brother—it doesn't matter. The idea is to allow someone else the honor of being *your* caregiver. Decide whether this is easy for you, or hard. The harder it is, the more it may be wise to practice, asking for more favors.

- Answer the following questions. If you come up with more than one "no" answer you might want to take some time to step back and re-evaluate your role as a caregiver.

  - Do you ask the person you care for what he or she wants and needs, versus assuming that you already know?

  - Do you generally refrain from helping or intervening until asked?

- Can you share with him or her some of your own wants and needs without feeling guilty?

- Can you name some of the gifts you presently receive from him or her—things you're truly grateful for?

---

IT MAY BE MORE BLESSED TO GIVE THAN TO RECEIVE, BUT THERE IS MORE GRACE IN RECEIVING THAN GIVING. WHEN YOU RECEIVE, WHOM DO YOU LOVE AND PRAISE? THE GIVER. WHEN YOU GIVE, THE SAME HOLDS TRUE.

*Jessamyn West*

## All Creatures, Great and Small, Can Give

Anna, who volunteers with her therapy dog Lizzy in a local children's hospital, told me an interesting story one day about giving, receiving, and healing.

A young girl had been grappling with cancer for months. She'd grown wobbly and weak, lost most of her hair, and lay in bed at home listless and deeply discouraged. She was surrounded by professional caregivers of the highest quality—nurses, doctors, specialists of various sorts, and so forth—all of whom brought their considerable gifts to bear upon her situation.

Nor was it just professionals trying to help her, but also family members, neighbors, friends, and teachers. Nobody liked to see her so sick. They tried to get her to eat. They brought her hugs and backrubs, toys and new books, bathrobes and slippers. Sadly, these caregivers—professional and personal alike—failed to make any significant impact. The child continued to weaken, day by day, until she was but a shadow of her former self.

One day, the child's grandmother brought the girl something different. It was a small, somewhat emaciated dog with a matted, clumpy white coat. "This dog needs a name and a home," the grandmother told her, setting it gently down on the bed. "She has been diagnosed with cancer, and her owners just left her at the vet. I told him that if he'd be willing to try some experimental treatments, we'd care for the dog ourselves. Do you think you could take this on? Of course the rest of us are willing to help, but most of the responsibility would be yours."

The grandmother was taking a big risk. What if the dog died in a few days or weeks? Would that leave this child in a state of more desolation than she could bear? What if the dog required more care and attention than its owner had stamina to give? What if she just didn't like the animal?

The child slowly reached out and took this pathetic bundle of fur into her arms. She began to whisper into its ear. At last she lifted up her head a bit, looked her grandmother in the eye, and said, "I think I can do it. Her name is Patchy, because her hair is all patchy. Just like mine." She smiled at her grandmother for the first time in months.

In the weeks that followed, the little girl took exquisite care of her new dog. She showered it with tenderness, offered it food but never forced it to eat, kissed it good-bye each time it went to the vet, and greeted it with open arms each time it returned. She talked to Patchy a lot, quiet words whispered into white fur—words that no one else could hear. Most often, the two of them could be found together, pressed somehow against one another.

Patchy's most vital quality was her willingness to receive what her new owner had to give. Patchy truly needed all this child's love and attention, and took it in freely, no strings attached. Likewise, the little girl received no long answers, no worried or fretful looks, no strained efforts to take the pain away—only rapt, silent attention and a cold nose on her cheek. No strings attached. And, slowly, the child began to recover.

When Anna finished her story, I found myself deeply curious about the outcome. "How did it all turn out? Did the little girl live?" I asked.

"The little girl kept recovering, until she was all better. Patchy lived for some months, and then died—but not before her friend had really begun to thrive."

"Do you still see the little girl?" I asked.

"I am the little girl," she said. And then, looking a little embarrassed, she added, "If you'll excuse us now, Lizzy and I have some hospital visits to make."

---

IN THE END, SOMETIMES, WHAT AFFECTS YOUR LIFE MOST DEEPLY ARE THINGS TOO SIMPLE TO TALK ABOUT.

*Etty Hillesum*

# A Father's Hard Lesson

My wife moved out unexpectedly while our sixteen-year-old son Jason was on a spring vacation school trip. He pulled up to the bus station and tumbled out with the others, only to learn that his mother was gone.

Things had been rough in our marriage for a pretty long while, but neither Jason nor I had anticipated this abrupt departure. I was left speechless trying to explain it to him because I didn't really understand it myself.

I did—somewhere deep inside—feel terribly responsible and terribly guilty. What more proof did a guy need that he was totally inadequate? It was a time for some harsh self-criticism, even self-hatred. It was a time of fear, hopelessness, and way too much preoccupation with what I had done wrong and how I had failed. Before long, all of this turned into an incapacitating depression, and I found myself in a therapist's office.

Jason didn't get depressed. Instead, he acted out. He started running with a different crowd of kids, skipping school, and things like that. Some nights he'd come home way after curfew, and I could tell he'd been drinking.

At first I thought he was going through a temporary thing that would eventually come to its own natural end. When that didn't happen, though, I got more and more worried. His mother had been largely in charge of rules and limits before, but now I was on my own. I laid down the law and then dished out the punishments in a vain attempt to control his increasingly wild behavior. Nothing worked. We fought and shouted and swore at one another. He walked out. I walked out. It was a big mess. Things only got worse.

Somehow, Jason made it through the school year without flunking out of school, but when summer came, all the free time was a major disaster. I hardly even saw Jason anymore. One night, I got a call from the police about some trouble he was in. Then, to cap it all off, he ran away in early July.

I was furious and underneath that, overwhelmed with grief. I had already failed as a husband, and now here I was failing as a father too. It seemed like more than I could bear. The empty house haunted me. Sleeping and eating were a real challenge. I was actually using Jason's behavior as proof (or disproof, in this case) of my own worth.

My therapist recommended that I try out "Parents Anonymous." Desperate, I went to my first meeting. This group of parents was not what I expected. They had all experienced some version of what I was going through. Many had lived through police arrests, running away, or a lot worse.

When it came my turn to talk, my story spilled out in tears as much as words. They listened quietly, and not a one of them told me what a horrible father I was. They just invited me to keep coming to meetings and assured me that I would continue to hear many stories similar to mine, and maybe even learn some new ways of making life better for myself.

I left that meeting knowing at last I wasn't alone. That in itself was a tremendous relief, like a boulder being rolled off my back. In the weeks that followed— meeting by meeting—I began to learn about doing things a little differently.

Maybe the most important thing I learned was that I could have a good life no matter what Jason, his mom, or anyone else around me chose to do. Just because he was mad at his mom for leaving, or confused and out of control, didn't mean that I couldn't enjoy my own life.

I began to notice sunsets and read good books again. I even started laughing at jokes. It was a whole new way of being for me. For the first time in my life I really began taking responsibility for my own happiness.

Jason was back again by the end of summer, run down, but still unwilling to quit drinking. With the help and support of other parents, I made my expectations clear, told him how much I loved him, and then, so to speak, let go of the back of the bicycle seat.

Gradually Jason began to see that his own gifts and strengths, not my parental interference, would have to see him through. He ended up going through a treatment program, getting off probation, getting his drivers' license back, finding new friends—basically, building a new life for himself. That was five years ago. He'll graduate from college next fall.

I have learned to love my son in a way that doesn't weaken or insult him. I'll always be there when he falls, but I won't hold the bike up. I've come to believe it's the best kind of care a loved one can give.

*Louis Thomas*

---

HERE I LIE

HAVING LEARNED THAT IN LIFE

THERE ARE BUT TWO THINGS:

LOVE, AND CONTROL.

NO ONE HAS BOTH.

*Inscription on a tombstone*

# WAY 8 :

# Learn to Say "No"

TAKING A NEW STEP, UTTERING A
NEW WORD IS WHAT PEOPLE FEAR
MOST.

*Fyodor Dostoyevski*

Dostoyevski was on to something. It is always challenging for us as human beings to take a new step, replace a familiar pattern with a new one, or speak a word previously unspoken. Often, for caregivers, one of the most difficult words to get out is the word "no."

This is for good reason. On some level, we have allowed increased concern and awareness for the well-being of another into our own hearts and lives. To say "no" when the stakes are low or the outcome insignificant, that's one thing. But to say "no" when other lives are involved, that is quite another.

This does not, however, make the word itself or its boundary-creating function unnecessary. As one of my colleagues pointed out the other day, "Sometimes you have to choose the smaller negative in order to allow for the larger positive."

"No," in other words, has its place.

There is the tale of a student invited to his teacher's house for tea. He loved his teacher and depended upon him for wisdom in all the ways of the world. He was indeed looking forward to a meaningful exchange.

"What lesson might you offer me today?" he asked.

His teacher said nothing. Instead, he began to pour tea from the pot into his student's cup. At first he filled the cup halfway. Although his student thought that would be plenty, the teacher continued to fill the cup. The tea rose all the way to the cup's edge and began brimming over. It spilled onto the table, and dribbled down into the student's lap, then sloshed onto the rug. Still his teacher continued to pour and pour, until wetness was everywhere.

"What are you doing?" the student at last cried out in confusion.

"No. What are you doing?" The teacher asked back. "Why did you not say 'no' to me? Why did you not tell me to stop?

"This is your lesson," the teacher went on. "Before you can grow in wisdom or empathy for others, you must learn one very important thing—how to say 'no' to too much. You must learn how to monitor the fullness of your own cup. Otherwise, you will continually find yourself in confusion and messiness. You will be distracted from your real work with others, simply trying to manage the overflow in your own life."

Although I first heard this tale years ago, I still, on a hectic day, return to the image of the overflowing cup. If I imagine my life as that cup, I can quickly become attuned to what it contains, how it is too full, and what I need to do in order to bring it into balance again. This is not for my well-being alone. It is for the well-being of others too. I have come to see that an over-full cup can take in little, including the wants or needs of loved ones.

When my life becomes over-full, it is time to say "no." This requires an assessment of what can be let go of and of what cannot. I simply cannot do everything, be everything, or achieve everything, no matter how much I want to. It is far more effective to accept my limits and work with them than to pretend that they don't exist and become flooded with frustration.

Our culture teaches us that saying "no" is simply not acceptable. Somehow, we ought to be able to do everything we set out to do. Isn't this the land where shoeshine boys can become President? Shouldn't we, as caregivers, be able to fulfill our tasks efficiently, if not effortlessly?

This attitude can both set us up to fail, and deprive us of our humanness. Of course we have to say "no" at times. Of course we can't do everything. To assume otherwise is a dangerous journey into denial.

Another way to look at it is this: every "no" is also, in some sense, a "yes." The student with the teacup, had he said "no" to overflow, would have been saying "yes" to a far more functional state of moderation. When I say "no" to an over-committed schedule, I say "yes" to a far more balanced and productive state of serenity.

Saying "no" to a big time commitment may be saying "yes" to more time for rejuvenation. Saying no to an unreasonable demand can mean saying yes to freedom from resentment or frustration. And the good news is this: saying "no" gets much easier with a little practice! It does not take long to learn that responsible use of this tiny yet powerful word allows for a caregiving approach that is much more liberated, joyous, and effective.

---

ONE CANNOT PUT A QUART IN A PINT CUP.

*Charlotte Perkins Gilman*

## Learn to Say "No"

- Reflect upon your life as a caregiver and write down the answer to this question: What is a commitment or task that you would like to say "no" to? Now, turn the page over, and write the answer to this next question: "If I were to say 'no' to this commitment, what would I be saying 'yes' to?" You might want to repeat this exercise a few times. The deeper your sense of how "no" can also mean "yes," the more free you may feel to say it.

- Start out the morning with ten beans (dried chickpeas or lentils, for example) in your right pocket. Throughout the day, move one bean from your right pocket to your left each time you'd rather say "no" but don't. By the end of the day, count the beans in each pocket. If you find more beans in your left pocket than you'd like, begin the next day by putting in your right pocket only the number of beans you are willing to "spend." For some people, especially those caring for highly demanding loved ones, this exercise can be both an eye-opener and a great reminder of when a limit has been reached.

- See if you can come up with one, two, or three commitments that you'd name most important and meaningful in your life. Condense each of these to a single word or phrase. Each one of these is a big "yes"—something you want to be intentional about supporting and nurturing. Carry these in your pocket, your purse, or at least your heart. Notice the ways in which your daily choices align with each big "yes." You now have a criterion for when to say "no."

SAYING "NO" CAN BE THE ULTIMATE
SELF-CARE.

*Claudia Black*

## What to Do With a Nest of Tools

Jan had known her husband since they were both sixteen years old. He'd laid eyes on her, known he wanted to marry her in an instant, and pursued her for the next several years.

She'd been a strong young woman, however, and careful to take her time deciding what to do. When at last she agreed to marry him, it was out of nothing less than a deep and abiding love for him. In other words, when Jan said "no" she meant it, and when she said "yes" she meant it as well. Thus had their marriage proceeded for over twenty years, including the sharing of a family business and the raising of two fine boys.

When Jan's husband was diagnosed with a serious, chronic illness, she knew in her heart that she was prepared to be his caregiver no matter what that entailed. Together they arranged for him to spend his days on a couch in the living room where others could visit him easily even if she had to be at work.

He had always loved to tinker with things and had a real gift for repairing appliances and other household items. Consequently, as the days went by, he gathered around himself a number of small tools, mechanical parts, and other items.

At first, this seemed like an excellent pastime for him. As time went on, however, Jan learned that it had a difficult side effect: it made a real mess out of the living room. Furthermore, the mess was growing, not shrinking. Her husband, unable to get up and put anything away, continued to gather around himself (with the help of well-meaning friends and visitors who wanted to make his life easier) so many items that Jan could barely enter the living room. Eventually, things got way out of hand. There were nuts and bolts on top of the television, screwdrivers and wrenches strewn across the coffee table, tubes of grease and glue, vises, squares, washers, engine parts, lengths of pipe, spools of wire, tacks, drills, and other odds and ends everywhere.

Finally she asked him to please begin picking up, offering to help herself. The condition of the living room was increasingly disturbing to her. He resisted. On some level, he seemed to take comfort from the "nest of tools" he had created.

Jan grew to hate the messy living room more and more. And yet, she felt she had no right to put her foot down. After all, why should her needs precede his? He was the sick one! And why did she care anyway? It was only some tools. Surely she should learn to simply tolerate this situation. Surely she should just practice getting used to it.

Despite such seemingly altruistic thoughts, Jan could tell that her "cup was over-full" with turbulent emotions: frustration about having no peaceful place to be with her husband in her own house, guilt about feeling frustrated, and anger about feeling guilty. She was finding less and less room within herself for other emotions that had far more power to heal and sustain: emotions like patience, generosity, and tenderness.

At last, Jan chose to say "no," even though it seemed like one of the most difficult things she had ever done. She found a way to tell her husband that this arrangement was simply too hard for her. She knew he needed things to do and tools to do it with, but at the same time she needed her living room in some semblance of order. How might they work this out together?

At first Jan's husband was hurt and angry, just as she had feared. He had lost so much to his illness already; did she have to take this away from him too? In a surprisingly short while, however, he came around. After all, he did love her, and he did want to honor her needs. They eventually worked out a compromise. He arranged as much of his "nest" as he could fit in a multi-shelved cupboard that she bought and then set up for him within reach of his place on the couch. Everything else was boxed and taken to the basement. She agreed to bring various items up to him if he really needed them and if he let her take something else down in exchange.

The real gift for Jan in all this was learning about what it felt like to say "no." In saying "no" she had emptied her cup of all kinds of unnecessary stresses and difficulties. She had used a smaller negative to affirm a larger and far more valuable positive. Once again, she was able to approach her husband with the honest, loving openness that had earmarked their relationship for decades.

---

IT IS NOT BECAUSE THINGS ARE DIFFICULT THAT WE DO NOT DARE; IT IS BECAUSE WE DO NOT DARE THAT THEY ARE DIFFICULT.

*Seneca*

# Tribute to a Grandfather

*The following story, told by a granddaughter at her beloved grandfather's funeral, is a poignant illustration of how to wield the word "no" with grace and wisdom.*

My grandfather taught me many important lessons.

I remember when we would visit my grandparents in Missouri I couldn't wait for the ride with Granddad in the pickup truck. We would go to the East farm and the North farm, and he would tell me all about what crops they were growing that year. Then to the West farm where there was a patch of land left to nature, and he would tell me how important it is to leave some of the land to the rest of the creatures we live with here on earth. Maximum profit is not as important as sharing the world with the other living things around us, he said.

He would talk about the land with pride. Money comes and goes, people come and go, but the land remains. It was here before us and will be here after us, so we should respect it.

I remember in college, at nineteen, there was something I "needed" that cost $50. More than I had. I don't remember what it was that I so desperately needed, but I do remember calling my grandfather. He never said "no" to me.

I explained my situation and asked if he would help me with the money to buy what I needed. He calmly said, "It is easy to confuse the difference between what we need and what we want. We need food, shelter, the basic necessities in life; the rest, we want. It is important to understand the difference between what we need and what we merely want. It is important not to take what we have for granted. For we will always want more."

I took that lesson to heart and realized whatever it was I thought I needed, I didn't.

About a month later I got a letter in the mail from my grandfather, sending me greetings and $50, no strings or explanation attached. I knew I didn't need whatever it was; I knew he knew I didn't either. But, he wanted me to not only have what I needed, but also have what I wanted.

I didn't want his lesson wasted. Instead of buying whatever it was, I spent the money on cookie ingredients that I brought to the local battered women's shelter and made cookies with some of the children staying there. Knowing the difference between what one needs and what one simply wants can be fussy in this culture; he taught me how to clear up the view.

Someone asked me to describe him long ago. I said, "He was patient, kind, and fair. He was always right, in my mind; he could do no wrong in my heart. He would always end a conversation with, 'I love you most.' I believed him."

Granddad, I love you the most too, and I'll miss you.

*Natasha Yates*

---

TO KNOW WHAT YOU PREFER INSTEAD OF SAYING AMEN TO WHAT THE WORLD TELLS YOU OUGHT TO PREFER, IS TO HAVE KEPT YOUR SOUL ALIVE.

*Robert Louis Stevenson*

# WAY 9 :

# Go With the Flow

YOU CAN'T PUSH A WAVE ONTO THE
SHORE ANY FASTER THAN THE
OCEAN BRINGS IT IN.

*Susan Strasberg*

Caregiving is *not* like making a soufflé!

You may wonder what this means, but the more I reflect on this piece of advice from my unconscious, the more it makes a lot of sense. Let me explain.

A soufflé requires meticulous attention. It has to be done just right or it collapses. No slogging in a dollop of this, an inspired pinch or two of that! The ingredients must be measured just so, the eggs beaten just so, the oven heated just so, and then the entire masterpiece whisked out to the table at just the right moment.

When all of this actually occurs as it should, the results are impressive. There is nothing quite like a large, beautifully puffed soufflé poised in the center of a well set table, its crust slightly brown, its steamy warmth aromatically filling the room. It is a clear indication that the cook is skilled, careful, practiced, and in full control.

Now you may understand when I say that caregiving, usually, is *not* like that. Those of us who bring strong control agendas to caregiving will often find ourselves in tears by the end of the day. We finally figure out how to give the pills in just the right amounts at just the right times, and the doctor changes half the prescriptions, requiring us to begin all over again. We plan a day away, knowing that we're in desperate need of a break, and find ourselves worrying about our loved one the whole time.

The skills that serve us best in caregiving are not control, mastery, and precision. They are more apt to be flexibility, ingenuity, forgiveness, and a willingness to surrender at the right moment. Caregiving is more like making a hearty stew out of things you find in the fridge. You take what you've got, do the best you can with it, put it all together in a spirit of love, and leave the rest in God's hands. A pot of stew may not be that dazzling on a beautifully laid table. But it doesn't collapse either.

Caregiving invites us to go with the flow. It can teach us a great deal about flexibility of both heart and hand. In this regard, I have always loved the Sufi story of the river's encounter with the desert. The river had been powerful and flowing for as long as it could remember. It had traversed mountains and plains, and across ice. Then, one day, it came to the desert.

At first it tried to cross the desert by pouring its waters as forcefully as possible out onto the sand. But the waters only sank in and disappeared. The river was terrified. Clearly, its old ways of getting where it wanted to go were not going to work here. It had no clue as to how to cross a desert.

After a long while, the river at last decided to ask the wind for some advice.

"You will need to relax, and let me lift you up," the wind explained. "If you allow yourself to become vapor, I will gladly carry you across the whole desert in a short time. Then you can become a rainstorm, tumble down out of the sky in the form of millions of raindrops, and become a river once again."

The river was shocked. "Vapor!" it cried out. "What is vapor? And what is a rainstorm? Raindrops? I can't become those things. I am a river!"

The wind tried to explain. "But you are many things. Yes, you are indeed a river, but a river and a cloud of vapor and a raindrop, though different, are really only different forms of the same thing. I would call this thing your essence, and I wonder if you have not forgotten about it."

"But if I am a river," the river said stubbornly, "how can I be something else too?"

"Trust me," came the wind's reply. "Try to trust me, and I will show you. You can be many, many things, without ever losing your precious essence, my friend."

The river, frightened and unconvinced, pondered the problem for a long time, but decided that there was no better choice. "I guess I am ready," it whispered to the wind at last.

The wind lifted the river up lovingly, urging it into the much lighter form of vaporous fog, and in a spirit of great tenderness carried it across the desert. All the while, it whispered words of comfort to the river. The river began to relax. And then at last the wind set the river down as gently as possible on the far side, and went on its way.

The river, for its part—having grown far wiser than before—flowed forth with a new heart, one open to far greater possibilities.

As a caregiver, I have often felt like the river did at first. I've wanted to do things my way. Usually, at such times, I have been motivated by fear of doing something wrong or by need for control. However, I have been taught by circumstance that flexibility, surrender, and openness will carry me far more effectively to my destination. I have learned that caregiving at its best is about going with the flow.

Caregiving—indeed—is *not* like making a soufflé.

---

IT IS POSSIBLE TO BEFRIEND UNCERTAINTY . . . TO REMAIN AWAKE TO ALL POSSIBILITY.

*Rachel Naomi Remen*

## Go With the Flow

---

- While slowly clenching your fists, ask yourself: "What is it that I have the strongest need to hold on to in my present caregiving situation?" Let the feeling of your tightening muscles help you discover what you never want to let go of. Grip your fists tight for as long as you can, all the while pondering what you want to hang on to. Now, begin to loosen your grip. Slowly let your muscles relax. Imagine letting go of what you have been clinging to. Feel the blood rush back into your palms, then your fingers. Release your tension, your hold, your determination to hold on. Relinquish it into the air, and into the hands and care of a loving God. Loosen your hands and with them your fear, your need to clutch or control, your focus on certain prescribed outcomes. Do this again if you'd like, this time inhaling as you clench, and exhaling as you release.

- Reflect upon a time in your life that reminds you of the river meeting the sand, a time when you encountered a problem you thought you'd never be able to get through. How *did* you tackle this problem? How did you have to change or adapt in order to find your way? Were there unexpected helpers that came along? Did you discover previously unknown gifts or strengths within yourself? What did you learn? Now, using the wisdom you gathered from that experience, write a letter addressing yourself (in second person) about your present caregiving situation. "Dear <u>insert your name,</u>" you might begin, "I know it's sometimes hard for you to go with the flow of these circumstances, but I trust you can find a way. Here are some things I've learned from tried and true experience that might help you. . . ." Find words to articulate those lessons from your past. Close your letter with an expression of love and encouragement, and sign it. Now do something rather unusual: mail it to yourself. Open it up when it arrives a few days later and read it anew.

- This is an excellent meditation for helping your whole body remember what it feels like to go with the flow. Once you have done it once or twice and learned the overall narrative, you can repeat this exercise any time. Read and reflect:

Imagine that it is autumn. Notice the deep azure of the sky, the brisk fresh breeze; feel the tingling coolness of the air. Relax, inhaling and exhaling deeply a few times.

Imagine that you are a leaf on a tree. You have lost much of your green, and become a beautiful collage of gold, rose, and bright orange. You are drying out, and the tiny place where your stem connects to the branch is becoming brittle. You watch your neighboring leaves all around you—letting go of the tree, floating and drifting down, down, down, and out of sight.

At last, it is your turn. You feel the slight wrench of the stem as it is pulled off in the autumn wind, and then you are on your way. You don't drop straight down, but dip and sway back and forth, gently slicing the air. There is nothing to do but relax, and follow the direction the wind is taking you.

Like many of the other leaves nearby, you land in a lazy, shallow stream that winds slowly through the field near the trunk of your tree, and into a beautiful wooded area. As you touch the stream, you realize that it is warm and fluid and gentle, and that where it will carry you is your true destiny. Your only choice is to allow yourself to drift along.

At first you try to resist, try to gain some control, but gradually you realize how fruitless this is. You have no arms to flail, no legs to kick, no voice to protest, no way whatsoever to do anything but follow the lazy current.

And so you surrender. As the stream carries you gently, smoothly along, you simply lie back and look at the sky, the branches arching overhead, the patterns of the clouds, the golden haze of the sun. You just lie back, and relax.

---

SAY TO YOURSELF: BE STILL. GROW QUIET. FOREGO FOR AWHILE THE ACTIVE TENSE. . . . NOW FEEL THE STEADY PULSE, THE WHEELING OF THE HEAVENS, THE RHYTHM OF DAY AND NIGHT . . . AND LISTEN LONG ENOUGH TO LET LIFE SPEAK TO YOU.

*Arthur Foote*

# A Garden Full of Wisdom

I love to cook. And that's what I do most often. I cook.

My husband Stan and I raised eight kids together, and for every kid for every birthday, I made a beautiful cake and a party meal. If I count all those birthdays up, it comes to 164 cakes and 164 meals. That's not even counting the sixty-two birthdays of Stan's that we celebrated together during the years of our marriage, or the sixty-two anniversaries we shared, or any of the birthdays of the grandchildren (we have seventeen of them) or great-grandchildren (we have seven of those, with another on the way!).

We have quite a clan here, and I still love to cook for all of them, even though I'm eighty-three years old. Every spring, I still plant a large garden in the backyard. I've done that for over half a century. And every fall I can pickles and pie fruits, tomatoes, sauces, and jellies. I reap what I have sown from the beauty and the bounty of God's earth, and it never fails to do my heart good. There is no greater joy for me than feeding my loved ones well.

Stan was my best fan when it came to appreciating my cooking, and it showed! Especially in later years, he developed a little pot belly from eating all my good food. He could hardly ever say no to a second piece of my pie, and after he retired, it just caught up with him. I teased him about it, but that didn't slow him down.

That's why I got a little worried, about three years ago, when he began to lose weight. He seemed to be eating just as much as ever, but he was growing thinner and thinner. And he seemed more tired and listless, too. I urged him to go to the doctor, but of course he put it off.

Finally he'd lost so much weight that I was getting frightened, and so were the kids. When we finally got

him in for an exam, the news was very difficult. He had
cancer, and it had metastasized. There was not going to
be a cure.

Stan was eighty-four when he got the diagnosis,
and I had just turned eighty. We had known that sooner
or later this would happen to one of us, but even so it
was a terrible shock. His health went downhill pretty
fast after that. Before we even had much chance to
adjust, the hospice folks had come in to help.

It was in the fall. We set up a hospital bed for Stan
in our living room. From there, he could look out the
bay window right into the yard. It was beautiful out
beyond that window. The leaves were turning, the
garden was withering, the sky was that bright deep
blue that colder weather so often brings with it. Stan
watched the birds gather in flocks to fly south. He
watched the pumpkins ripen, and the first snowfall.
Many days, I sat in the rocking chair next to him, and
watched too as winter came, and wrapped everything,
in pure clean white.

More often, though, I was in the kitchen. It stood to
reason that with Stan not feeling so well, I should cook
him exactly what he wanted. For a few months there,
he seemed to be drawing a lot of strength from what I
made him. I fixed all the comfort foods: sweet
puddings, delicious hot soups, fresh crusty breads,
casseroles filled with meats, vegetables, and noodles.

I will always remember those few months as a
special time. It's hard to watch someone you love so
much begin to fail. You want to do everything you can
for them. You want to somehow make everything better.
It felt to me like feeding Stan was going to do that, make
everything better. In my head, I knew that didn't make
any sense. But in my heart, I couldn't help myself. And
so I cooked and cooked and cooked, and he ate and ate
and ate—all the way into the middle of winter.

Some time after we had celebrated Christmas and enjoyed a quiet New Year with all the family around and some unforgettable champagne toasts, Stan began to lose his appetite. I'd bring him a big bowl of soup, and he'd only be able to get down a few sips. He'd ask for a slice of my famous cherry pie, and set the dish down after a bite or two. I would always urge him to try to eat a little more. It just seemed to me that food was the stuff of life; that in order to live, he needed to eat. And eating was my specialty. If I cooked something delicious enough, if I spent enough time on the right recipe, surely he would keep eating for me.

I smile at myself in retrospect, but at the time, I was only doing what I thought best. The more Stan lost his appetite, the more I tried to get him to eat. Several times a day I'd come to him with some lovingly prepared foods, urging him to try a sip or a bite or a nibble. Sometimes he would give something a try, and then throw it up later. Sometimes he would just close his eyes as though he was exhausted.

Finally, one day in early spring, our kindhearted hospice nurse sat me down for a talk. All fall and winter, she had been coming to help us several times a week. On that day, she told me something that was hard for me to hear.

She told me that it was natural for a dying person to gradually lose his appetite and stop eating. And she also told me that she thought Stan was trying to eat my food so he wouldn't hurt my feelings. That's why he was throwing up more, because he was pushing himself in order to show me that he loved me by eating my food.

She and I talked about what it would be like for me to stop feeding him. It would, I told her, be like depriving him of air to breathe. Again, she gently repeated that dying people naturally lose their appetite.

"But look at the garden," I said to her, tears coming into my eyes. "Look at how the beans are coming up, and how the tomatoes are beginning to ripen. Are you telling me that this year Stan may not be able to eat any of the beautiful fresh vegetables I've grown for him?"

She put her hand on mine. "Yes, I am telling you that. You can keep pushing him to eat, and he'll probably keep trying, out of love for you. But it is hard on him. Believe me, it is harder for him to eat now than it is for him to refrain from eating."

I broke down in sobs. This was much too hard. After sixty-four years of gathering so much satisfaction from cooking for this dear man I loved so very much, it was time to stop. I didn't know what I would do with myself. The hospice nurse stayed and tried to comfort me as best she could.

"You know, a garden is beautiful in more ways than one," she said. "I bet Stan would draw a great deal of pleasure from simply watching your garden grow out the window. And when something gets ripe, you can bring it in to show him. He might find great pleasure in holding it or smelling it even though he no longer wants to eat it."

The hospice nurse was right. Stan did enjoy watching the garden grow and me bringing a big, red, ripe tomato or a juicy cucumber in for him to look at. He'd hold it in his palm, feel its heft, hold it to his nose as though it were a bouquet of flowers, and say, "Beautiful job, Mother, you've done it again!"

As I cooked for him less, I sat beside him more, holding his hand, reading, or just gazing out into the yard. Those were our last days together, and they were more precious to me than I could ever say. Stan died peacefully in the middle of summer. He had not eaten in over a month. Somehow, I had managed to find new ways to express a love that was very old and deep.

But don't get me wrong. I'm back at the stove now, busy as ever. I've got plenty of kids and grandkids, and they come over a lot—just to see what's cookin'. Of course, this brings me great joy, as it always has. But I've learned something too: The cooking isn't the love, it's only a sign of the love.

*Annie Burroughs*

---

THEREFORE I TELL YOU, DO NOT BE ANXIOUS ABOUT YOUR LIFE, WHAT YOU SHALL EAT . . . WHAT YOU SHALL WEAR. IS NOT LIFE MORE THAN FOOD, AND THE BODY MORE THAN CLOTHING? AND WHICH OF YOU BY BEING ANXIOUS CAN ADD ONE CUBIT TO YOUR SPAN OF LIFE?

*Gospel of Matthew*

## In a Different Place, and in It With Her

When we move into the realm of caregiving for the terminally ill, or when we are caring for someone with a life-altering disability, we walk through the wall of so many taboos. Suddenly we are allowed to think about death, about limits, about transgressions. Society finally allows us to cry in public, to feel overwhelmed, even to tell our grief to strangers.

But other taboos remain, of course. For me, the largest taboo was the day I realized that I wished my daughter would die.

How conscious this wish was is debatable. I remember thinking, "Well, when she has this surgery for her teeth, perhaps she will have a reaction to the anesthesia, and maybe she won't survive, and perhaps that will be the easiest thing for all of us."

I never thought the words "I wish she would die." I just thought, "Maybe it would be easier if she weren't living."

This thought did not keep me from checking and double-checking her medication with three different hospital anesthesiologists. The thought did not keep me from pacing the halls anxiously, wishing that I smoked cigarettes, because if I did, I would have smoked six at once. And the thought did not keep me from weeping with gratitude at her bedside when she came around, bloody-mouthed, dazed, and trying to claw out her IV. She looked like a small Greta Garbo with her short light hair brushing her now even higher cheekbones, her pale skin, her big blue eyes.

How, then, did I come to wish that her life might end?

My daughter has severe autism. She does not have speech as we know it. She is considerably larger than her peers, and strong. Her strength and her sensory overload and her frustrations that we will never understand have caused her to be dangerous to herself and others when she runs into the street and breaks windows and grabs necks. She has been hospitalized many times: on my fortieth birthday, on New Year's Day, in the middle of the summer. The medications and therapy appointments and doctors' appointments and administrative phone calls on her behalf are endless—a sensation familiar to any caregiver.

One thing I have come to understand is a simple fact that, like all simple facts, is enormously complex. When I told a family doctor about the wish I had that my daughter not come out of anesthesia, he told me: "That was a natural thought. You want the pain to end. You want her pain and your own pain to end. Who wouldn't want pain to end?"

He helped relieve my guilt a bit, though I still think he was going easy on me. And I told him there was something else I had wanted with that wish: I had wanted to find a way to mourn—completely, neatly, totally.

But then I remembered something about my father's death four years before. I am still mourning the loss of him, and I still don't know how to put his death or his life in perspective. In other words, even death could not solve the yearning to mourn completely, neatly, and totally. Death may put an end to the doctors' appointments, but it doesn't put an end to the sorrow or the frustration or the anger or the fear or the expectations or the love.

I must have realized some of this when my daughter came out of the anesthesia. When she came around, I felt like I was passing through into a new phase with her. Some subtle shift was easing into our relationship: a renewal, a chance, something. I was shedding expectations that I would know how to feel, and how much to feel, and what to do with those feelings. I held her, and knew that I knew nothing about what to expect or hope or dream.

And I can't close this reflection by saying, "But I did know one thing, and that was. . . ." Because there was no one thing that I knew at that moment. I was just in a different place, and I was in it with her. It was me, her, and love.

*Elizabeth Burns*

GENTLE ME, HOLY ONE, INTO AN
UNCLENCHED MOMENT,
A DEEP BREATH, A LETTING GO OF
HEAVY EXPECTANCIES,
OF SHRIVELING ANXIETIES, OF DEAD
CERTAINTIES . . .
THAT SURROUNDED BY THE LIGHT
AND OPEN TO THE MYSTERY
I MAY BE FOUND BY WHOLENESS.

*Ted Loder*

# WAY 10:

# Be Gentle With Yourself

---

YOU HAVE TO TAKE CARE OF
YOURSELF. IF YOU DON'T TAKE CARE
OF YOURSELF, YOU WON'T BE ABLE
TO TAKE CARE OF ANOTHER
PERSON.

*Dorothy Calvani*

I am not particularly fond of flying in airplanes, but I have come to appreciate the part where the flight attendant tells you about how to use the oxygen masks. You know the message, I'm sure. Generally speaking, it is the always the same: if there's a loss of air pressure in the cabin, put your own oxygen mask on first—*before* you try to help anyone else with theirs.

This bit of advice first captivated me as a young mother. I was preparing for take off, holding a tiny new infant in my lap, when the pre-flight instructions began. The idea of helping myself before tending to my baby seemed shocking to me until I realized that without oxygen I'd pass out and would probably never get around to the baby at all.

If you are caring regularly for a loved one, self-care is as important for you as oxygen. Without it, you may—in a shorter time than you might expect—be unable to help anyone. I'm not sure why this is, but caregivers as a group—no matter what their age, gender or circumstance—are notorious for ignoring self-care.

In my work as a hospice chaplain, I even discovered a medical term for it: "caregiver breakdown." Caregiver breakdown is a real diagnosis applied to those who literally exhaust themselves caring for the hospice patient in their charge. A person diagnosed with caregiver breakdown is eligible for greater insurance coverage, more respite services, and increased nursing and home care support. The condition is taken that serious.

My aunt who cared for my grandmother unceasingly for months was hospitalized with an ulcer on the day my grandmother died and was unable to be present at the funeral. My friend's mother, caring full-time for a husband with Alzheimer's and convinced that she could do no less, ended up "sending" him to a nursing facility by having a heart attack and becoming so disabled that there was no other choice.

More than merely being aware of your own needs, caring for yourself means remembering that you are one of God's precious creatures, doing some of God's precious work, and then treating yourself accordingly. It's an invitation for you to be more than tolerant of yourself, but truly gentle and loving with yourself as well.

In some cultures self-care is both highly valued and understood as inextricable from care of others. Author and speaker Martin Prechtel describes the Tutuhil Mayan culture, for example, where such mutual care has highest priority.

Among Tututil Mayans, it was taboo for anyone to endure sorrow or difficulty alone. This means that if a person looked sad as he or she walked down the road or expressed discouragement while speaking to a friend or neighbor, others would immediately gather around the person. Not next week, not tomorrow—immediately. Wherever the person was when this happened, others would stop, encircle him or her, and help. They didn't try to figure out if the troubles were justified, or if the person brought suffering on himself or herself. They gathered quite simply to help. If you were a caregiver among the Tutuhil Mayans, impending discouragement or exhaustion would be immediately tended to. Caregiver breakdown would never occur.

Granted, the Tutuhil Mayans are an ancient, small, and tribal culture. Even so, I cannot help but ponder the wisdom of their ways in terms of sheer survival. There is a deep truth in the understanding that we are all part of one another and that whenever one of us is helped, all of us are helped. Whenever the caregiver is helped, the one cared for is helped.

This means you should never forget to care for yourself. Notice when you need help, and be sure to find it. Notice when you are weary, and be sure to do whatever it takes to regain your strength. When you are sad, seek comfort. When you are confused or at a loss for what to do, invite counsel. Consider it not a luxury but an imperative: be gentle with yourself.

---

TO HAVE THAT SENSE OF ONE'S INTRINSIC WORTH WHICH CONSTITUTES SELF-RESPECT IS POTENTIALLY TO HAVE EVERYTHING . . . TO LACK IT IS TO BE LOCKED WITHIN ONESELF, PARADOXICALLY INCAPABLE OF EITHER LOVE OR INDIFFERENCE.

*Joan Didion*

# Be Gentle With Yourself

- Find a comfortable place to reflect and write. Close your eyes and invite into consciousness one single image or symbol for good self-care. Often, when I'm feeling stressed, I'll imagine the oxygen mask dropping down in front of me, waiting for me use it. Find a personal image of your own. It might be an oxygen mask, a big flower, a sparkling lake, or a pillow. After the image has come to you, describe it in writing. Capture as many details as you can. Elaborate, if you want, by writing down special meanings you ascribe to it. Make it as real, as memorable, as clear, as possible. Use the image when you are tempted to abandon self-care. Call it up to help you make a good decision.

- H.A.L.T. This handy acronym comes from a twelve-step program. The letters of H.A.L.T. stand for Hungry, Angry, Lonely, Tired. Use H.A.L.T. as a way of monitoring and remembering good self-care principles. If you feel rundown, HALT. Take a minute to ask yourself four questions. Am I hungry? Am I angry? Am I lonely? Am I tired? If you can say "yes" to any one of these, do something about it before continuing with your day. If you can say "yes" to more than one of these, you've probably gone too far already, and tending to your own needs is more important than ever.

- Take yourself on a weekly date. Think of what you'd like to do for fun. Then ask yourself on a date. Write this date in your appointment book like any other, and try not to hurt your own feelings by canceling out at the last minute. Excursions to restaurants, museums, zoos, public gardens, therapeutic massage, movies, paths through the woods, lectures, concerts—all these are possibilities.

---

DON'T ASK WHAT THE WORLD
NEEDS. ASK WHAT MAKES YOU COME
ALIVE, AND GO DO IT; BECAUSE
WHAT THE WORLD NEEDS IS PEOPLE
WHO HAVE COME ALIVE.

*Howard Thurman*

# The Official Care Team Strikes Again . . . and Again

No doubt you've heard the African saying, "It takes a village to raise a child." In my opinion, it would be just as accurate to say, "It takes a village to care for anyone in need."

Believe me, I learned that the hard way.

I am not married, and I have no children. Over the past few years, as my mother got into her mid-eighties and needed more help, it just seemed that I was the best choice of her three kids to provide it. I'm a consultant. I generally keep my own schedule, so I had the added advantage of job flexibility. My brother and sister were both trying to raise kids, save for colleges, and keep large households up and running. They just didn't seem to have time like I did: to share meals with her, get her to the doctor, and just in general enjoy being with her.

My mom and I talked about the best way to work things out and decided that she should move in with me. I love Mom with all my heart, and we got off to a great start together. About three months into this, I developed what seemed like some kind of sinus infection and didn't waste too much time getting to a doctor. It seemed like a small problem, and I came home with some antibiotics. Little did I know how quickly everything would get out of hand.

I can hardly describe the months that followed. At first the doctors thought I had some kind of allergic reaction to the antibiotics. I was having a terrible time breathing and ended up in the emergency room. When the breathing problems refused to go away, they thought it might be asthma and treated the condition as such.

For some reason—still unknown, by the way—I then entered into a crippling bout with acute pain and stiffness in my joints, which seemed to be some kind of arthritis. It continued to be one thing after another. Each new affliction seemed a mystery, and the connections between different symptoms continued to baffle a large team of doctors.

As crazy as this may sound, eventually my mom and I inadvertently switched roles. She had come to my home to be cared for, but I needed more care than she did. So, despite her own painfully stiff joints, she took to tottering around the kitchen to try to bring me meals, keep things clean, whatever was needed.

My mom and I were a disaster waiting to happen, but I just kept pushing and pushing myself. She couldn't drive, and eventually I couldn't either. At the time, that felt like the final blow. Actually, it turned out to be the beginning of the solution.

We both needed help getting to appointments now, and money was running through my fingers at a terrifying rate. Had I been able to afford a taxi, I certainly would have used one for both of us, but I couldn't. I had to resort to calling upon friends to get us places. I tried to spread the favors out, never asking one person twice in a row. And I tried to never complain, which meant that I avoided giving anyone the whole story about how much my mom and I were struggling.

After a few months of this, my friends got together for coffee one Saturday morning. I couldn't be there myself, but somehow the matter of my health came up. As they talked, each one chipping in something different about what kinds of favors I'd been asking, a big picture slowly emerged for them. I guess they finally saw—probably better than I did at the time— how much trouble my mom and I were really in.

They say that when you're in trouble you learn who your friends really are. Well, I did. And I still cry just thinking of how good they are. Don't ask me why or how, but by early afternoon that same Saturday they were knocking on our door. My best friend, Susan, said, "Hello, Marie, let me introduce you to your new 'Official Care Team.'"

I was shocked. All this time I'd been worried about asking too much from any one of them. It never occurred to me to ask for help from all of them together—as a group. That was their idea. They had made a list of what they thought Mom and I needed. Next they designed a schedule and a way for sharing the load. Between all of them, it really wasn't too much. Teamwork made the load bearable and, according to them, fun.

Each day for the following month, they told me, they were going to take turns cooking, cleaning, and driving for us. One was going to come in and give us a weekly massage. Another, a pastor by profession, was going to lead the others in a weekly prayer effort.

They had thought of everything. They taught me more about taking good care of myself than I had learned on my own in an entire lifetime. I was so relieved and so touched by their kindness that I sat down on the couch and just sobbed.

Their efforts probably made the difference between keeping Mom at home or putting her in a care facility, the difference between me getting through this crazy symptomatic time with my health, or risking some chronic snarl of problems.

After a month of loving care, I had just about returned to my former self. Mom was cheerful and rested. As for my "Official Care Team," they seemed in great shape too, not to mention downright proud of themselves—as well they should have been.

At this point, I have great hope that I can continue to be Mom's primary caregiver. I am meticulous about self-care. But my main strategy for being good to myself these days is to let others help me when I need it. The fun part is this: my friends and I have realized that we can all be the "Official Care Team" for one another. This means that if Susan ever gets sick, the rest of us are committed to helping her. Same with Janice, Libby, Joan, Anne, or Beth.

We know from experience now—we're good at it!

*Marie Sanford*

---

MAY THE HAND OF A FRIEND ALWAYS

BE NEAR TO YOU;

MAY GOD FILL YOUR HEART WITH

GLADNESS TO CHEER YOU.

*Anonymous*

## The Guys Who Love Their Wives a Lot

No matter how forgetful I may grow over the years, I hope I will never forget the "Guys Who Love Their Wives a Lot." I met them at an assisted care facility during my year of residency as a chaplain. At first, they were not the "Guys" so much as a dispersed collection of individual men. They had something important in common, but they had not yet discovered it.

It's common knowledge that women in our culture tend to live longer than men. So, among married couples, women are more apt to be end-of-life caregivers. It also means that in facilities designed to serve our seniors, the majority of residents are usually female. Statistics, however, are not everything.

I have witnessed many situations in which a wife's health begins to fail first, at which time her husband will enter lovingly and with deep dedication into the role of caregiver. Because this is less common, however, it also tends to be less recognized. As a result, husband caregivers often have trouble finding men in similar situations. They are apt to feel isolated in their role. Many of their friends are still being cooked for, cared for, by an attentive wife. These men, by contrast, do all caregiving and household chores themselves.

This particular facility was set up so that spouses could live with one another as long as possible, the stronger often caring for the weaker until this was no longer viable as an option. Here, as in most cases, the majority of couples were comprised of women giving care to their husbands. But in about six units of this facility's one hundred and fifty, it was the other way around.

The six dedicated male caregivers in this facility had never met one another. Each one spent his days caring for a fragile or confused spouse, and there was little time for more.

A nun who came on a weekly basis to offer communion and prayer first noticed these men and their particular isolation. Not one to dwell for long in inaction, she immediately invited all six of them to a special Bible Study Group—for men only.

"But I'm Protestant!" one said.

"Doesn't matter," she answered. "Come anyway. You're going to love it."

"But how can I leave my wife for an hour? She's too confused!" another said.

"We'll get help from the staff," Sister said curtly, though not without tenderness.

And so they had their first meeting. They studied that passage from the book of Ruth:

> Do not press me to leave you and to stop going with you, for,
>
> wherever you go, I shall go,
>
> wherever you live, I shall live.
>
> Your people will be my people,
>
> and your God will be my God.
>
> Where you die, I shall die
>
> and there I shall be buried.

These six men had a great deal to say about this passage. They knew, in a deep way, about the ramifications of it. They knew what it meant to literally embody the kind of fidelity it described. As they spoke and reflected together, each one of them quietly noticed something significant: all of the others understood the meaning as well.

Sister closed the hour by saying, "Praise God! You guys certainly love your wives a lot. But if you don't spend some time enjoying life in your own right, you're going to run into trouble. I expect you back here next week, same time. Come, you're going to love it."

The next week, they were all there. After a few months, they started having lunch together when their Bible Study was done. They could be picked out of the crowd in an instant: six guys with gray hair, plaid shirts, and suspenders; six guys with rough laughs and caring hands, eating sandwiches together at a single table, their caregiving conversation interspersed with fishing memories, hunting lore, and fond stories about their grandchildren.

Before long, they began coming up with schemes for going out together. One time, they went off to play bingo. Another time, they went to a baseball game together. And once they went off to a bar together and played a few rounds of poker.

Always, they kept their trips short. Always, they made sure their loved ones were not left alone. Just as dependably, though, they allowed themselves a good time. They seemed to understand how much their own well-being mattered—how much a few hours of fun could help them fulfill their primary obligations.

Gradually, they came to be known as the "Guys Who Love Their Wives a Lot." Everyone knew that it was because they loved their wives a lot that they had learned to be this intentional about preserving their own sense of joy.

One day near Christmas they were having their usual lunch together when some staff members approached them carrying six identical packages gaily wrapped in red and green. They were caught off guard. As they began to open them, however, they shook and roared with laughter.

The staff had ordered, specially made, six bright red T-shirts. And across the front of every T-shirt, in bold black print, it read: "Guys Who Love Their Wives a Lot."

---

IF I AM NOT FOR MYSELF, WHO WILL BE FOR ME?

*Talmud*

# Let Humor Heal You

AT THE HEIGHT OF LAUGHTER, THE
UNIVERSE IS FLUNG INTO A
KALEIDOSCOPE OF NEW
POSSIBILITIES.

*Jean Houston*

The *St. Paul Pioneer Press* publishes a regular column entitled "Bulletin Board," in which readers share true stories about their own life experiences. Some years ago, as I lay slumped on an old sofa, grieving the loss of a beloved aunt, I came upon the following submission:

> I had the misfortune to have to attend the funeral of a very wonderful woman who'd died very unexpectedly. The church was full to its capacity with people who had come to pay their respects. It was at a time when the song "Wind Beneath My Wings" was very popular, and it had been selected as a song to be played during the funeral—right after the oldest grandson had delivered a eulogy he was unable to finish because he was so choked up.
>
> Well, the time for the music came, and whoever was operating the record player dropped the

needle on the wrong spot. The church was filled with "Under the Boardwalk." People had been crying so hard before, during the eulogy, that it went immediately to tears of laughter. You could see people's shoulders quivering because they couldn't help but laugh.

I remember thinking, from my glum spot on the sofa, that I shouldn't laugh at this article, and that the people at the funeral shouldn't have laughed either. I sat there with the newspaper in my lap, arms folded, lips pressed together, trying to maintain some semblance of what I considered a more appropriate and sober attitude.

But I couldn't. In spite of myself, I found the laughter bubbling up from somewhere deep inside. Perhaps you've heard Chuckles the Clown, on the old Mary Tyler Moore show, talk about "a little song, a little dance, a little seltzer down the pants." Well, much to my chagrin, I seemed to have a little seltzer-down-the-pants. Pretty soon I was giggling, then guffawing. At last I surrendered, and simply let joy happen. And I can honestly say, in ample retrospect, that my deceased aunt would have probably laughed as well.

What a tremendous relief! It seemed as though all the sorrow and tensions, all the anxieties and worries of recent days were being dissolved and washed away by this sudden flood of laughter.

Laughter is a symptom of joy. And joy, whether in the form of laughter or just a quietly happy heart, mysteriously heals, energizes, and uplifts the human spirit all at once. This has been known for centuries. As far back as the 1600s, physician Dr. Thomas Sydenham said, "The arrival of a good clown exercises more beneficial influence upon the health of a town than twenty asses laden with drugs." And in recent times, far more measurable scientific research has proven his comment to be true.

Granted, sometimes the circumstances surrounding a caregiving situation don't seem funny. And if you just don't feel like laughing or even smiling, it's impossible to force either. However, we can be open to letting laughter happen if and when it fits. So, keep your eyes open for joy in unexpected places because it can be so healing, so lifegiving, for both you and your loved ones.

If you'd like to observe the healing powers of humor, try watching the movie *Patch Adams*, starring Robin Williams. What Dr. Patch Adams seemed to understand so well (and what many of us under stress so easily forget) is that there are two ways to approach a difficult situation. One way is to focus on the difficulties and invest all your energy in trying to reduce them. The other is to focus on something besides the difficulties, thereby giving them less space in your overall life.

One viable way to deal with the difficulties in any given situation is to reduce the proportionate space they consume in your day, by allowing joy to crowd them out—not entirely, of course, maybe just a bit more as time goes on.

Gareth Branwyn, one of Patch Adams' own patients, had endured excruciating back and joint pain since adolescence due to arthritis. Branwyn tried every traditional and non-traditional therapy he could find—all to no avail. Dr. Adams, in the initial interview, asked Branwyn not what his symptoms were, not what his treatments had been, but this: "What is your passion in life? What turns you on? What motivates you? What excites you?"

Branwyn found himself disturbed by this approach and this eccentric caregiver who invariably chose to focus on positives first. But it all came clear to him one evening later on, as the two of them sat together before a stunningly beautiful sunset. The sky was emblazoned with orange, and so breathtaking that neither patient nor doctor could even speak. After a long while, Adams turned to him and quietly whispered, "Do you have arthritis while you're watching this?"

As Branwyn wrote later, "The question absolutely floored me. 'No, come to think of it, I don't.'" For the first moment in a long time he had completely forgotten his own suffering. The joy of what lay before him had proven more engaging. By nature incompatible with desolation, it had, for a little bit, simply crowded out his chronic pain.

As a dedicated caregiver, you deserve your own share of beautiful sunsets, bouts with pure joy, eruptions of wholesome laughter, doses of humor, and excursions into sheer happiness. And so, perhaps, do those you care for.

---

THERE AIN'T MUCH FUN IN MEDICINE, BUT THERE'S A HECK OF A LOT OF MEDICINE IN FUN.

*Josh Billings*

## Let Humor Heal You

- Sink into a good chair with your writing tools nearby. Ask yourself the last time you experienced a full and lifegiving sense of joy. Perhaps you were laughing at a joke or stifling giggles about an absurd situation. Maybe you were, like Patch Adams and his patient, gazing at something wholly beautiful. The main thing is: can you remember it? Can you remember how it affected your body and spirit? Pick a favorite memory. Now write it down: the circumstances, what happened, and how it affected you. After writing, allow yourself to bask for a bit in the glow of what you have just described. Happiness is potent not only as an experience, but also as a memory.

- Give yourself a few moments to notice how thoughts and their actual content have an affect on your whole system. Read the following words to yourself slowly from left to right, as though they are a sentence:

GLOOM DESPAIR MELANCHOLY DARKNESS TEARS HARDSHIP LOSS SORROW SADNESS ANGUISH DREAD TORMENT PAIN TROUBLE FEAR FRUSTRATION REGRET MISERY REJECTION

Stop and ask yourself: "How do I feel?" Now try these words, reading them in the same manner:

JOY CHEERFUL MERRIMENT JOKING GIGGLES SILLY LAUGHTER CHERISH FUN GLADNESS JOLLY HILARIOUS PLAYFUL EXUBERANT PLEASURE BRIGHTEN ENERGIZED AMUSEMENT GENTLE WARMTH

How do you feel now? Often, while reading the first list, people will express becoming more and more rounded in the shoulders, tense in the muscles—in general just more acutely sad. The second list, on the other hand, often brings about a very different—and more hopeful—state of body and mind, functioning almost like an antidote.

- If we expose ourselves to humor, we'll likely catch a bit of its healing power. It can be "caught" from watching the right movie, reading the right book, or even listening to a certain bit of music or recorded dialogue. When you go to pick out a rental movie, try the comedy aisle once or twice. Walk down the joke book aisle in the bookstore. Or as you sip your morning coffee, check out the comic section in the newspaper.

---

START EVERY DAY WITH A SMILE AND

GET IT OVER WITH.

*W. C. Fields*

## Grandma Gets Us Going

My grandfather was diagnosed with diabetes shortly after the Great Depression. He had taken a number of very serious financial losses, and the doctors felt that probably his system succumbed to the terrific stress of that situation, making him more prone to chronic illness.

Diabetes was a newly diagnosed condition back then, and treatment methods were crude compared to what we have today. My grandfather never went to work again after his diagnosis, and his daily care regimen was all-consuming.

My grandmother, his primary caregiver, went at the task with distinctive love and passion. For the next thirty years or so, she boiled insulin needles to sterilize them, prepared three meals each day that were carefully designed to keep his blood sugar under control, and helped him with the urine tests that would monitor his glucose levels. She was always there to give him the orange juice that would pull him out of insulin shock, day or night, and she was there too as he experienced the long term complications of this ravaging disease: loss of eyesight, neuropathy, and later on, confusion, uncontrollable infections, and so forth.

It would have been easy for her to become depressed under this kind of sustained stress. And yet, what I remember most of all about my grandmother was her ebullient sense of humor. Hearing her laugh was an engaging constant in my childhood. She would erupt into gale upon gale of giggles until she had to set down her knitting, wipe her eyes, and literally scold herself into a more serious demeanor.

Sometimes jokes would set her off, sometimes small daily events or stories. Sometimes, she would set up a bit of mirth herself by executing some merciless stunt with my grandfather's false teeth or putting on one of her famous costumes. I have many memories of her coming around the corner of the house to surprise us, having sneaked out the back door dressed as a clown, a strange lady with a gigantic hat and a beard, or some other character of her own creation.

Sometimes, though, even serious situations got her going. I remember one time in particular when my grandfather, an avid pipe smoker, rose up from his resting place on the couch in that state of confusion so much a part of his later years and wandered out the door without telling anyone. When we realized he was missing, we knew enough to fear for his well-being and organized quickly into a search party. Combing the house and the yard, we did not succeed in locating him.

We regrouped and set out again. This time, I found him. He had wandered to the edge of a nearby woods, probably unaware of where he was, and had fallen down a steep embankment. He was lying motionless on his back at the bottom.

Terrified, I ran home and got the grown-ups. A small group of us—my grandmother included—returned to the place I had seen him. Before we could find out if he had any broken bones, my grandmother began to giggle. I remember my uncle turning to her with an angry expression on his face. Her giggles, thus censored, turned into gasping squeaks and snorts, making it hard for her to even speak.

Finally we saw what she was pointing and snorting at: it was his pipe. Still locked firmly in his teeth, it continued—absurdly—to emit a thin curl of white smoke from its well-worn corncob bowl. My grandfather—not hurt after all—had wandered out the door, walked at least the length of a block, fallen down a long hill, lain there—and not once stopped smoking his pipe!

"George, dear," she whispered, kneeling down beside him and putting a tender hand on his cheek, "tell me then, how is your pipe?"

"Just about out of tobacco, I suspect," he said, as though he were speaking to her from a chaise lounge on the patio. This set her off again, and she muffled guffaws, snorts, and chuckles all the way home.

My grandmother, bless her soul, taught me how to embroider, deep fry homemade doughnuts, and make a good bed. But most of all, she taught me—without even trying to—about the healing, lifegiving power of a good laugh or two. I will be forever grateful.

---

He who laughs, lasts!

*Mary Pettibone Poole*

## Getting My Head Unstuck

Comedian Roseanne Barr once said, "There's a lot more to being a woman than being a mother, and there's a lot more to being a mother than most people suspect."

As a single mom of two, I have a sneaking suspicion she's right. There are times when I am more exhausted than I ever thought possible; more frustrated than I ever dreamed I'd get; and more confused about what is right than I'd ever want to admit in public.

Fortunately for me, both of my children have this odd knack for doing something unpredictable and dear at just the right moment (that being the moment before I really lose it)—some little word or gesture that reminds me yet again to laugh, to appreciate life, and to focus on what's really most important. My friends tell me I experience these moments because of how I look at life, but I'm pretty sure it has more to do with God's sense of humor. Let me give you some examples of the kinds of thing I mean.

One recent morning, after a harrowing breakfast comprised of far too many spilled juices and airborne Cheerios, I had finally managed to get my son Ben out to the car, and buckled into his seatbelt for the drive to school. Just as I was thinking about how hard this all was—how much directing kids is like herding cats—Ben turned to me, looked lovingly into my eyes, and said, "Let's roll, babe!" (Who cares about herding cats, if they're that sweet?)

Another time he and I were struggling in one of those endless lines at the grocery store, cart full to the brim, when I realized I'd left the cash at home. "Oh Ben," I exclaimed in frustration, "I can't believe I forgot the money. I must have lost my head!"

"Oh no, Mama," he said, wanting to help me out, I guess. "Don't worry, it's still stuck right there on top of your neck."

I'm supposed to feel bad after a line like that?

When Ben's little sister Annie arrived, needless to say, the complexity of our days increased. He so wanted to share his room with her. After much deliberation, I invited him to go shopping with me for a little crib or bassinet we could set up near his own bed. "That's okay, Mama," he assured me, "she can just sleep on top of me."

Sweet, sweet boy. He brings me more joy than I can tell.

Annie in her own right brings more joy into our home than a human being may rightfully deserve. She has a special fondness for music that will surface unexpectedly and make my own heart sing, no matter how tired or frustrated I am. Once when a certain tune came on the radio, she was filled with an excitement that had no discernible source. "What is it, Annie?" I asked her. She explained, "Oh, Mama, can't you tell? That song goes perfect with my dress!"

How I wish I could experience the world as she does.

Just the other day, she indulged in some mild form of naughtiness and was told to take a timeout in the living room. I set the timer for ten minutes, and just after that, her beloved older cousin Libby arrived. Ben, Libby, and I were chatting in the backyard, when I was very surprised—no more than a minute or two later— to hear the timer going off in the kitchen.

I peeked in to find Annie beeping an extremely accurate imitation of my oven timer. She just couldn't wait to see Libby! I released her from the timeout early, with points for creative problem solving.

I guess that's what my children teach me about: creative problem solving, particularly as it relates to fresh perspective, joyous abandonment, and the millions of ways life's doldrums can be outsmarted.

Without Ben and Annie, true, I'd be less tired, less stretched, less worried, less spent, and less frazzled. Surely, though, I'd also be far less aware of the ways God's holiness can infiltrate and illuminate even the smallest moment.

Bless their sweet little hearts.

*Kimberly Lund*

YOU GOTTA KNOW HAPPY AND YOU
GOTTA KNOW GLAD, CAUSE YOU'RE
GONNA KNOW LONELY AND YOU'RE
GONNA KNOW SAD.

*Mark Knopfler*

# WAY 12:

# Remember the Future

---

IN THREE WORDS I CAN SUMMARIZE
EVERYTHING I'VE LEARNED ABOUT
LIFE: IT GOES ON.

*Robert Frost*

At first glance Robert Frost's three-worded wisdom—"it goes on"—sounds obvious and logical. Of course life goes on.

Even so, what may be obvious and logical to the mind is not always quite so obvious and logical to the heart. When you're changing the diaper at midnight, having just changed it a few hours ago and a few hours before that, and a few hours before that, it is easy to feel like you're going to be changing diapers forever.

When you're at the bedside of a loved one, listening to them struggle to breathe, you want to breathe for them, but you can't. Their struggle for air seems endless; the sound goes on, and on, and on.

At times like these we tend to think back on the day when we didn't even know how to change a diaper. We remember with longing a time when our loved one's breathing was so effortless and easy as to go unnoticed. In many cases, a caregiving situation will evoke the past. Sometimes we remember old times as easier,

145

healthier, or simpler days. No matter what details or emotions we conjure up, however, the general direction of our thinking tends to be backwards. We think of what has now, for better or worse, come to an end.

And sometimes, without meaning to, we overlook the quiet truth that this particular caregiving situation, no matter what it may be, will someday come to an end as well. We can be certain that the one or ones we care for today will not be with us forever. They will grow up and move away, or regain strength and health, or die, or require a different caregiving setting, one in which our role has been radically changed or diminished.

And even if they change very slowly or very little, we will be changing. We might need to move away or become unable to provide what we had before. For that matter, we might die.

A day will eventually come when we will have experienced the end of caregiving, one way or another. On that day, we will likely look back in a spirit of reflection, contemplating if we did what we really wanted to do, asking ourselves if we accomplished what we set out to accomplish, and wondering if we followed our own heart and our own values in the matter.

Too often, I have witnessed, among those looking back, a disturbing sense of regret. Too often, I have witnessed guilt or sorrow that has no simple means of resolving itself. I have heard litanies of "If only I'd . . ." or "How I wish I had. . . ." This is why I have come to believe that as caregivers we need to remember not just the past, but also the future. Granted, we need to cast the wide nets of contemplation behind us to capture all the precious memories and life lessons there. Also, though, we need to cast our nets forward in time, toward days we've yet to see. We need to remember the future: remember that it inevitably awaits all of us, and that one day it will be called the present.

For many years the co-ministers of the church I attended in Minneapolis closed every worship service with a benediction that ended like this: "So let us be about the task; it is for today, and for times we shall never see. The materials are very precious, and they are very perishable. Amen." These words offer an eloquent summation of what it means to remember the future. They remind us that the present moment is fragile and changing, and that we give it integrity by dedicating it not only to today but also to times that lie ahead. It is for our own sake, for the sake of our children and our children's children.

It is for the sake of our world.

---

MY INTEREST IS IN THE FUTURE . . .
BECAUSE I'M GOING TO SPEND THE
REST OF MY LIFE THERE.

*Charles Kettering*

## Remember the Future

- Settling into a quiet place, gently invite yourself to imagine a time in the future, a time when your caregiving role has ended. Simply pick one scenario that seems likely or desirable to you. Notice how your surroundings have changed, how your daily life has changed. Notice how it feels: the ways you are sad, the ways you are relieved, the ways you are at peace or content. Write a reflection that begins like this: "Looking back I am very grateful that as a caregiver, I. . . ." Describe the things you did, the values you embodied, the choices you made, that you especially appreciate from this vantage point.

When you are finished, allow yourself to drift back to the present moment once again. Ask yourself if you are helping to create, at this time, a future that you will be at peace about and grateful for.

- Ask the one you are caring for, as well as other involved family and friends, what they "can hardly wait for" or what they look forward to as they move into the future from this present situation. Then, just listen. Try not to influence or critique their responses. Let them tell you about their hopes, dreams, and needs; let their words inform and influence you. The future is co-created by everybody.

- Draw upon "tombstone wisdom." Ask yourself the following questions: "What would I want written on my tombstone? What is it that I most want to be remembered for? What trait or quality—when all is said and done—will be the one I hope to have embodied during the course of my life?" Keep it to a sentence or two, and know that eventually it may well be written in stone. For now, though, inscribe it on a piece of paper—or upon your heart.

---

THE MOMENT MAY BE TEMPORARY

BUT THE MEMORY IS FOREVER.

*Bud Meyer*

## Surviving My Own Mistakes—Barely

You know, as I look back, I do kind of wonder how I got through the midlife stretch at all. Well, I barely did.

My husband Joe had been killed in a tragic and devastating car accident when I was thirty-six. At that time our son, Joey Jr., was ten, and our twins, Stella and Lila, were eight. This terribly painful event threw me into a long period during which I rarely planned more than a few hours ahead—much less a day, a month, a year, or a life phase.

My husband and I hadn't expected anything to happen to either of us. Our finances and legal matters were in naïve disarray. When he died, everything became a chaotic mess, touch and go all the time. I was just juggling things at breakneck speed, and there seemed to be no time left for anything except the basics: laundry, food, earning money, taking care of the house, helping kids with homework, car repair, driving people places, new shoes and school clothes, sports, dance lessons, and on and on. Believe me, I felt desperate around the clock, like a woman submerged in deep water who only on rare occasions could manage to make it up for air.

I'm not sure it needed to become a lifestyle, but it did.

I got so used to life careening along like a roller coaster that I guess somewhere in there I just stopped wondering about ways to slow it down. Sure, our clothes were wrinkled half the time, and we had a lot of peanut butter and jelly sandwiches for dinner, but we were getting by, and that was pretty much all I had come to expect.

When Joey graduated from high school, he got a scholarship to a good college, and off he went. To be honest, I didn't stop to think about missing him much. I cringe to say it now, but I'm pretty sure that on some level I was just plain relieved to have the kid-count go down from three to two.

Though there was every indication that Joey was happy and successful in college, he didn't call home much. He also didn't come home summers. I didn't stop to ask myself what that might mean. There would be one less mouth to feed, and things seemed generally okay. That's what I noticed.

Two years later, when the twins graduated, they too left home to head off in their own directions: one to a community college out of state and the other to the same college her brother attended.

To be honest, during those final years raising the kids, I was like a horse headed for the barn. Even though I was exhausted from all that I was doing and never really allowed myself to let up, deep inside of me, I was just waiting for the day I would be done. Just waiting.

This was never a particularly conscious thought, I would add. In fact, I was largely unaware of its depth and breadth in my life. It usually only reached consciousness in the form of brief expectations or anticipations, little wisps of thought that began with the phrase, "Well, when I'm finally on my own again . . ." followed by a sigh, a slump, or a tattered daydream.

In the fall of my forty-ninth year, for the first time in as long as I could remember, I was finally on my own. All the kids were finally gone. On any given weekday I could get up to a neat house and head off for a mere eight hours of work—no overtime, at last. Upon returning home I could mix myself a drink, put my feet up, watch the evening news undisturbed, fix a dinner of whatever I chose, read books for as long as I wanted, and go to sleep in perfect peace and quiet. I had achieved it at last: heaven on earth.

It was about three months before I began falling apart. In four months, I was so immobilized by depression that I got fired from work. I spent the fifth month in the psychiatric unit of a hospital, trying desperately to choose life over suicide. The sixth and seventh months involved a very slow recovery, a stretch at a halfway house, and a return home. It was a year and a half before I returned to work.

In retrospect, I can honestly say that this period of coming apart turned out to be one of the most meaningful and important phases of my life, though I would never, ever want to go through it again. The lessons may have been tremendously fruitful, but they were extremely painful at the time.

Now three years later I am just figuring out how to articulate those lessons. There are only two biggies, I think, but if I were to put them in some kind of order—an order of increasing importance, let's say—I'd do it this way:

*First, slow down enough to show love to your kids while you have them.* It wasn't that I didn't love mine. It's just that when Joe died like that, I stopped showing it in any real way. Sure, they saw me running around like a chicken with its head cut off, trying to do things for them. But they never heard me say how much I loved them. They didn't get hugged much, or kissed goodnight. We never spent an hour or two just goofing around together, having a good time. They never lingered at the kitchen table with me, telling me all about their fears and loves and passions. I was too intent on whisking the dishes into the dishwasher and starting the washing machine.

When my kids left, they stayed away. They didn't call. They didn't come home. They had come to experience me as someone who distanced them emotionally most of the time. What would be the point of calling home?

Believe me, those terribly painful months following their departure were very much about how deeply I did miss them after all, and about a thousand sudden regrets. Part of my therapeutic process, in fact, included making amends to them from the bottom of my heart and asking them for another chance.

Joey and Lila have expressed a cautious willingness to create a new relationship with me. Stella has not. I hurt my kids badly. I didn't mean to, but I did. Now, I live with the consequences of that. Every time Joey calls, every time Lila stops by, my heart flies into my throat with joy. And I grieve the absence of Stella almost as much as I grieve the death of her father. Maybe things will turn around later on. Maybe they won't. I've had to accept that.

*Second, don't ever lose yourself, no matter how hard that gets.* Whatever happened to me in all this? To put it simply, I lost myself. When Joe died I had some serious grieving to do. Instead of allowing myself to do that openly, I threw myself into frenetic activity. Ostensibly that was all for the kids. On a deeper level, though, it was a way of avoiding my own pain—distracting myself from it.

The problem was, in distracting myself from my pain, I also distracted myself from my *self.* By the time those kids left the house, I knew plenty about what I was tired of, what I didn't want to do anymore, what I could hardly wait to finish.

Get this, though: I didn't know anything at all about what I *did* care about, what I *did* love to do, what I *was* interested in, where my life *was* headed. I was a bundle of negatives.

You can't guide your life on negatives forever just like you can't drive a car backwards without eventually smashing into something. I no longer knew who I was. I had lost the big picture. I had sacrificed the past and, even more important, I had sacrificed the future—in order to focus on whatever moment, whatever need, whatever crisis shoved itself in front of my nose. When I was finally left alone, I was lost. Nothing around me but ghosts, regrets, and loneliness.

Meet the new me. Every morning, I light a candle for my beloved husband Joe, and I say a prayer for him, and spend some time talking to him about whatever comes to mind. There is so much I was never able to say to him. The wound after all these years is raw and sore, and only now just beginning to heal.

I have switched to a new profession—because I love it. Every day, as a teacher's aide, I help kids. In some way, I hope to give back to the world what I failed to give to my own kids—a loving, attentive adult who cares. I look forward, one day, to holding a grandchild.

I know what else I love: trips to Hawaii (am saving for the second one right now), flower gardens (planted twenty more bulbs last week), McDonald's hamburgers (politically incorrect, maybe, but I can't help it), good mystery books (headed for the library again this afternoon), and all sorts of other things that make life worth living in the long run.

There is no rush. There is no crisis. The future awaits me, thank God, and I will never again act as though it doesn't exist.

*Martha Mitchell*

---

REMEMBER THE LITTLE THINGS, FOR ONE DAY YOU MAY LOOK BACK AND REALIZE THEY WERE THE BIG THINGS.

*Robert Brault*

## And Last, Remember Your Holy Shadow

My friend and colleague Reverend Shelley Dugan has served for many years as chaplain in a nursing home. Her work there has made her sure of something our culture tends to deny: that all people, no matter what their age, demeanor, attitude, or condition, have profound gifts to offer. Even though she takes on a formal "caregiver role" at work, she has no illusions about how much she gains from those she serves.

Shelley has grown used to encounters with those who simply can't fathom how she, a caregiver, is also a grateful receiver at the nursing home. In order to illustrate her meaning, she tells a compelling story:

Once there was a woman so kind and loving that all the angels in heaven asked God to give her a magic wish, that she might be even more content and fulfilled in the future. God wisely suggested that they consult her first, that perhaps she did not want to receive such a wish.

It turned out that God was right.

This kind woman was content with life just as it was, and gently refused the offer. When the angels persisted, however, she said, "Very well then. As I move into the future I ask for this: that I may do a great deal of good without even necessarily knowing about it."

The angels, perplexed by her preferences, wanted to honor her request. At last, they designed a plan.

The woman's shadow, falling behind her and therefore out of her sight, would be given great power in the world. It would be able to cure disease, soothe pain, ease sorrow, and bring great joy to others. The woman herself would simply go about her life, her shadow following along silently behind her. Unbeknownst to her, though, everything her shadow touched would receive great bounty in terms of comfort and healing. Over the years, the woman's given name was forgotten. This is because everyone who came to know her simply called her the "Holy Shadow."

Shelley goes on to point out that, as far as she can tell, the residents in her nursing home all seem to have Holy Shadows. Without trying, without noticing, and most often without being acknowledged—just by being there—each one has a bounty of wisdom and experience to offer. To simply be with any one of them—to be gently brushed by the shadow of their presence—is to gain something.

I would posit that each of us—caregivers and caregiven both—has a Holy Shadow. Each of us offers healing in ways we're completely unaware of. So, why not be open to the most fruitful possibility of all: that each of us has something to give, and will always have something to give, wherever we go and whether we know it or not?

There is really only one thing that we'll need to follow us into the future: the Holy Shadow that is uniquely ours. To bring it along is paradoxically effortless. To trust in its presence, a little harder. And sometimes, to see it in others, a little harder still.

But it is there. It stands for all that we have to offer in the way of help and healing, often in spite of ourselves and our more conscious choices.

As we ponder our future, we should remember that literally everything upon this earth is more mysterious and rife with hidden holiness than we can ever know.

And that includes you.

---

MAY GOD BLESS YOU AND KEEP
YOU.
MAY GOD BE KIND AND GRACIOUS
UNTO YOU.
MAY GOD'S FACE BE MADE TO
SHINE UPON YOU
AND BRING YOU PEACE.
AMEN.

*Traditional blessing*

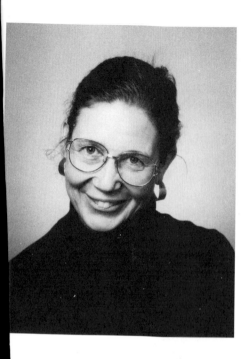

ained Unitarian Universalist minister,
hompson is a part-time chaplain working
medical center and a home health care and
ncy. She holds a Bachelor of Arts from
lege and a Master of Divinity from United
Seminary, Minnesota.
been a writer-in-residence at United
Seminary and The Ragdale Foundation,
Illinois, and her previous books include
and *Souls Magnified*.
resides with her family in Minneapolis,
s recently named Woman of the Year for
on achievements.

## ACKNOWLEDGMENTS

The story by Natasha Yates about her grandfather (Chapter 8, "Learn to Say No") is used by permission of the author. Copyright Natasha Yates, 2000.

The exercise in word boxes from Chapter 11, "Let Humor Heal You," is adapted from an exercise in the chapter "Jest 'N' Joy" in *The Wellness Book: The Comprehensive Guide to Maintaining Health and Treating Stress Related Illness* by Herbert Benson, M.D. (Simon and Schuster, 1992).

An ord
Gretchen T
with a large
hospice age
Carleton Co
Theological
She has
Theological
Lake Forest,
*Slow Miracles*
Thompso
where she wa
her social acti